# Solving Life's Problems

Arthur M. Nezu, PhD, ABPP, is professor of psychology, medicine, and public health at Drexel University. He is an elected fellow of the American Psychological Association, the Association for Psychological Science, the Society for a Science of Clinical Psychology, the Society of Behavior Medicine, and the Academy of Cognitive Therapy. Currently a trustee of the American Board of Professional Psychology, he served as president of the American Board of Cognitive and Behavioral Psychology, the Association of Behavioral and Cognitive Therapies, the Behavioral Psychology Specialty Council, and the World Congress of Behavioural and Cognitive Therapies. Dr. Nezu has contributed to over 175 scientific publications, is a consulting editor for numerous psychology journals, and a grant reviewer for the National Institutes of Health. He is also a practicing psychologist for over 25 years.

Christine Maguth Nezu, PhD, ABPP, is professor of psychology and associate professor of medicine at Drexel University. She has contributed to scores of scientific publications, has presented extensively at professional conferences around the world, and has participated on the editorial boards of leading psychology journals. Dr. Maguth Nezu is board certified in cognitive and behavioral psychology and is currently president-elect of the American Board of Professional Psychology. She serves on the board of directors of both the American Board of Cognitive and Behavioral Psychology and the American Academy of Cognitive and Behavioral Psychology. Her clinical research has been supported by federal, private, and state-funded agencies and she has served as a grant reviewer for the National Institutes of Health. She is a practicing psychologist for over two decades.

Thomas J. D'Zurilla, PhD, is professor in the department of psychology at Stony Brook University. He has published a number of pioneering theoretical and research articles on social problem solving, stress and coping, and problem-solving therapy. Together with Art Nezu and Albert Maydeu-Olivares, he has also published a self-report measure of social problem-solving ability, the *Social Problem-Solving Inventory-Revised*. His writings and measuring instrument have been translated into Spanish, Japanese, Chinese, German, and French. Dr. D'Zurilla is a member of the American Psychological Association, the Society for a Science of Clinical Psychology, the Eastern Psychological Association, and the Association of Behavioral and Cognitive Therapies. He has also been a practicing clinical psychologist for more than three decades.

# Solving Life's Problems

*A 5-Step Guide to Enhanced Well-Being*

Arthur M. Nezu, PhD, ABPP

Christine Maguth Nezu, PhD, ABPP

Thomas J. D'Zurilla, PhD

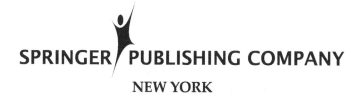

SPRINGER PUBLISHING COMPANY

NEW YORK

Springer Publishing Company, LLC
11 West 42nd Street
New York, NY 10036

*Acquisitions Editor: Sheri W. Sussman*
*Production Editor: Emily Johnston*
*Cover design: Joanne E. Honigman*
*Composition: Apex Publishing*

07 08 09 10/ 5 4 3 2 1

---

### Library of Congress Cataloging-in-Publication Data

Nezu, Arthur M.
  Solving life's problems : a 5-step guide to enhanced well-being /
Arthur M. Nezu, Christine Maguth Nezu, Thomas J. D'Zurilla.
    p. cm.
  ISBN 0–8261–1489–x
  Includes bibliographical references and index.
  1.  Problem solving. 2.  Life skills.  I. Nezu, Christine M.  II. D'Zurilla, Thomas J.
III. Title.

BF449.N49 2006
153.4'3– –dc22

2006018592

---

The problem is not that there are problems.
The problem is expecting otherwise
And thinking that having problems is a problem.

—Theodore Rubin

It's a troublesome world,
All the people who're in it,
Are troubled with troubles
Almost every minute.

—Dr. Seuss

# Contents

# Contents

# Solving Life's Problems

# CHAPTER 1

# Why You Should Read This Book

Low at my problem bending,
Another problem comes.

*—Emily Dickinson*

Are you feeling down in the dumps, sad, blue, like there's a cloud over your head? Are you feeling stressed out, tense, upset, concerned about the future? Are you having difficulties at work, finding it hard to get promoted, finding it hard to get a job? Are you searching for the meaning of life? Are you having arguments with your kids, parents, siblings, friends, or neighbors? Is your marriage unsatisfactory; are you having difficulties talking to your spouse? Is sex satisfying? Are you lonely? Looking for a meaningful relationship? Do you still get enjoyment out of your hobbies? Do you feel stuck? Are you having problems losing weight, quitting cigarette smoking, or maintaining a healthy lifestyle? Are you experiencing difficulties in adhering to the advice your doctor prescribed in order to deal with your heart problems or diabetes? Are you having difficulties making a tough decision about your career? A new job? Getting married? Having another child?

Should we go on? Anybody reading this book is bound to answer "yes" to at least one of the above questions. So what! Don't we all have problems? Of course! But why should *you* read this book? We wrote this self-help guide for people who experience *continued* difficulties in tackling these problems, who try, but are often unsuccessful in coping with many of the day-to-day hassles and strains, and who might find themselves worse off after trying to resolve one of life's problems. We wrote this for people who might not understand where they went wrong, why they failed, or why stress seems to just get the better of them. We also wrote it for those individuals whose lives are relatively stable and going well, except that their physical health is suffering and life just continues to interfere with their best efforts to adhere to their doctor's

1

recommendations about medication, exercise, or developing other healthy lifestyle habits. We also wrote this book for people who have adapted relatively well up to this point in their lives but are currently dealing with a problem that is either very complex, intense, or novel. Do any of these situations sound like what you are experiencing? If so, then that's why *you* should read this book.

## WARNING: THIS BOOK CAN CHANGE YOUR LIFE

Our journey through life certainly produces constant challenges. Moreover, as Emily Dickinson noted in her poem quoted at the beginning of this chapter, it sometimes seems like problems never end. Such problems include the common snags and obstacles that stand in the way of our dreams, or the unexpected personal demands that occur when we least expect them. Some problems originate from our relationships with others, such as family members, fellow workers, neighbors, and friends. Problems also occur when we continue to behave in ways that we would actually like to (or need to) change. On the other hand, problems can occur because others behave towards us in insensitive, uncaring, selfish, or hurtful ways. Sometimes our problems and the problems of those near to us have more to do with an unexpected situation, such as sickness or accidents. Conversely, some of our problems come from the inside and exist because of our own vulnerabilities, such as fears, anger, sadness, and regret. In all likelihood, most problems are caused by a combination of these types of factors.

One fact we know for certain is that life *is* full of problems. But more importantly, learning how to cope with them is extremely important to our mental health and physical well-being! For example, psychologists and other health professionals have been scientifically studying the consequences of unsuccessful coping for decades and have found that ineffective problem solving is strongly linked to the following:

- Depression
- Anxiety
- Suicidal thoughts and behavior
- Marital problems
- Child-rearing difficulties
- Alcohol and substance abuse
- Poor health habits
- Aggression
- Difficulties adhering to medical or healthy lifestyle prescriptions
- Difficulties managing chronic illness
- Worry

- Poor academic performance
- Poor work habits
- Negative physical symptoms (for example, elevated blood pressure, menstrual pain, back pain)
- Posttraumatic stress disorder

On the other hand, *effective* problem solving has been found to be associated with optimism, hope, greater self-esteem and self-confidence, improved health and emotional well-being, and a strong sense of overall life satisfaction. Effective problem solvers view problems more as opportunities for growth or positive change rather than threats, have self-confidence in their ability to adequately tackle difficulties, and attempt to react to problems in a thoughtful, planful, and systematic manner, rather than trying to go for the quick fix or avoid dealing with problems. These *effective problem-solving skills* serve to increase the likelihood that such individuals can adapt more successfully to life's strains and difficulties.

More importantly, decades of scientific research have found that training individuals in these effective problem-solving skills can have a significant impact on one's overall health and emotional well-being. This is the major purpose of this book—to teach people to become better problem solvers when dealing with life's difficulties. The techniques and tools for coping provided in this book can be applied to all of life's problems. These guidelines are based upon a particular type of counseling or life skills training that has been developed over several decades of clinical research known as *Problem-Solving Therapy*. Some of the areas of difficulty that have been shown through scientific studies to improve with this type of counseling include stress; depression; anxiety; suicide; various behavior problems; marital and relationship difficulties; health conditions such as cancer, diabetes, and chronic pain; and preventing relapse regarding substance abuse and obesity.

As such, this book is for anyone and everyone, for any type of problem, at any point in one's life. It can be read and used on its own; as part of a group discussion in your support group, community center, mosque, synagogue, or church; as a method to use in parenting or to work out marital and family problems; or as part of an individual counseling or therapy experience.

We have been talking about problems in living. Before we continue, let's define what we mean by a problem, as well as an effective solution.

## PROBLEM

Problems can be a single event or situation, such as forgetting your wallet after going off to work. They can also be a persistent series of related events, such as having continuous arguments with your spouse, difficulties relating to co-workers, or continuous financial strains. Problems can also involve deeper or more complex issues, such as being afraid of having intimate relationships, having chronic back pain, or experiencing an inability to overcome grief related to the loss of a family member.

In essence, problems represent a discrepancy between your current state (what is) and your desired state (what I want). This discrepancy is a *problem* because of the existence of various obstacles that block the path when trying to reach your goals. Given this definition, the same situation might represent a problem to one person, but because of different circumstances, it is not a problem to another individual. Usually, situations that serve as obstacles to goal attainment (that is, why a situation is a problem for a given person) include the following:

- Novelty or unfamiliarity ("I'm not sure what to do.")
- Complexity ("This is very complicated.")
- Conflicting goals ("I'm confused about what to choose.")
- Skill deficits ("I can't do that because I don't know how.")
- Lack of resources ("I don't have enough time to take care of that.")
- Uncertainty ("What's going on?")
- Emotional difficulties ("I'd rather do nothing because I'm afraid to try and fail.")

Now that we have defined what a problem is, what is an *effective solution?*

## SOLUTION

A solution is a person's attempt to either (a) change the nature of the situation so that it no longer represents a problem to him or her (that is, obstacles are overcome and goals are achieved), *or* (b) change one's own negative reaction to those types of situations that cannot be changed. For example, consider Bob and Paula, who are experiencing significant marital difficulties. If they both wish to solve such problems (that is, to improve their marital relationship), then possible obstacles to overcome may include poor communications, differing child-rearing philosophies, conflicting values, limited financial resources, and so forth. Our problem-solving guidelines would then be geared to help Paula and Bob overcome such obstacles in order to improve their marriage. However, consider a somewhat different scenario—Bob would like the marriage to continue, but Paula firmly believes that whereas

Bob "is a good friend, I no longer love him, our goals in life are so far apart, and I cannot see myself staying in this marriage—unfortunately, I think we got married too soon after we met and it was a mistake." If Paula continues to feel this way, then Bob's solution can no longer be one where he is trying to "maintain the marriage and get Paula to fall in love with me again," but one where he needs to "accept that my marriage is over and be able to go on with my life." This is a very important point—some problems can be changed and you should try your best to solve them by changing the situation in some way (for example, overcoming obstacles). However, if the problem is not *changeable,* than it is more important to try to change your reaction (grief, depression, anxiety, anger) in order to enhance your well-being, rather than maintain the unhealthy state of distress. In addition, because most of life's problems are complex, it is likely that often our goals for resolving a problem or adapting to stress would entail *both* types of goals, that is, some change *and* some acceptance.

Further, an *effective* solution, in addition to reaching either of the above goals, also is one that (a) maximizes positive consequences, and (b) minimizes negative consequences. It is one thing to overcome obstacles—it is quite another if in doing so, you either reap additional benefits or actually cause some negative consequences. This will be described in more detail when we talk about how to make decisions (Chapter 7).

We defined what a problem is, as well as what an effective solution is. You might now be wondering—how do problems and problem solving fit into my overall well-being? The relevance of trying to solve problems in living is contained in a model of stress and its effects on our health and emotional well-being that has been developed over several decades.

## PROBLEM SOLVING AND STRESS

Simply being human means that we all experience problems. In fact, we experience problems on a daily basis. Most of the time, these daily problems are small, like running late, for example, losing our keys, or not having exact change for the bus. However, sometimes we experience daily problems that are more significant, such as difficulties with our boss or coworkers, not having enough money to pay for the mortgage, or arguments in our relationships. Even though some of these problems appear small at the moment, over time if they continue, such smaller problems can create a lot of stress! As such, we are better off if we are able to resolve them early on before they begin to accumulate.

Life, unfortunately, presents us with bigger problems as well. These involve major life events that can have a negative impact on our overall quality of life, such as losing a job through downsizing, getting divorced or ending a meaningful relationship, experiencing the death of a loved one, failing at an important task, or becoming ill. These types of major events can often create additional smaller problems, which in turn make the original major problem even worse. This situation is often referred to as *stress*. For example, experiencing a relationship loss can easily change a person's life—people who experience such loss consequently also experience emotional distress, physical symptoms, concerns about the future, a change in their overall activity level, other relationship problems, financial difficulties, and so on. These additional problems can leave us feeling worried, sad, withdrawn, or irritable, and lead to other major problems or incidents such as loss of other relationships or serious problems at work. It is important to remember that *both* types of situations, that is, daily problems and major life events, can lead to stress.

## A DEFINITION OF STRESS

We often hear or read that stress is bad for us. But is this true? Before answering this question, we should explain what we mean by stress. Most people think about stress similar to the way we described it in the previous section, that is, the large and small pressures we are under and the problems we face. Behavioral scientists refer to this part of the overall stress process as *stressors,* or the stressful events that we experience. How we *react* to these stressors with our thoughts, feelings, and behavior is an important second part of stress. It is important to understand that *stress* is the result of the *stressors* (problems and demands we face) in combination with the way we *react* to these problems. This is an important definition to remember because, if we can't change the number or intensity of stressors that we confront, we can change our reaction to these stressors. If we react in ways that create more stressors, then we *increase* our stress. On the other hand, if we react to stressors with effective ways of coping, then we can *reduce* stress.

## NEGATIVE EFFECTS OF STRESS

If we think of stress this way, the answer to the question "Is stress bad for us?" is a resounding *yes*—excessive negative stress leads to both harmful emotional and physical consequences. Whereas some stress is good for us, as it helps us to stay alert and motivated, excessive stress can result in emotional difficulties (for example, strong feelings of sadness, worry, or anger), as well as affecting our physical health. Stress also leads to problems in the way we think, for example, having thoughts of failure, being confused, or having trouble making decisions without second-guessing ourselves. Our behavior often changes with increased stress, causing some of us to feel tired, fatigued, and avoidant, or others to become hyper-aroused, agitated, aggressive, and impulsive. With so many changes in our bodies and minds, it is not surprising that stress has been found to be a significant risk factor for various health problems, such as cardiovascular disease and stress-related immune disorders. Research has documented that emotional distress, such as depression, anxiety, and anger, related to both acute and chronic stress, can serve as risk factors for the initiation of a disease, as well as the worsening of existing problems. For example, emotional distress has been linked to increased elevated blood pressure, lower back pain, migraine headaches, asthma, gastrointestinal problems, increased blood glucose levels, lowered heart rate variability, and compromised immune functioning. It is not surprising, then, to learn that *decreasing* the negative effects of stress can:

- Improve your overall quality-of-life.
- Foster better mental and physical health.
- Help you make desired behavioral changes.

That's what problem-solving coping is all about! By being an *effective problem solver,* you can reduce the negative impact of stress. This program will teach you to use a five-step approach to solving life's problems as a means of enhancing your well-being.

## WHY A BOOK ON PROBLEM SOLVING AND NOT ONE THAT PROVIDES SOLUTIONS?

Wouldn't it be wonderful for us to be able to go to a sourcebook whenever we have a problem and look it up in the index in order to find *the* solution? Unfortunately, life is not like that, where one solution solves a problem for all who experience it. Each of you reading this book is an individual. Even if you are experiencing a similar problem as others, such as relationship difficulties, each person's circumstances are different. In fact, the reason *why* you might be experiencing relationship problems can be very different than the reasons why someone else might be having the same concerns. Just remember the last time a friend or family member tried to give you unwanted or incorrect advice about a problem that he or she experienced that was similar to yours. You probably thought—"Well, that solution may have worked for you, but I'm different!"

For us to try to tell you *what* to do to solve a given problem would be to deny the many differences that exist among people. In addition, if what we were saying before is true, that is, life is full of problems, then we would constantly be going to that sourcebook and not having time for anything else. As such, think of the following old wise saying as the underlying philosophy of this guidebook:

> Give people some fish, they eat for a day....
> Teach people to fish, they can eat for a lifetime.

In other words, having the ability to effectively solve life's problems allows you to continue to be nourished and enjoy enhanced well-being.

## ABOUT THIS GUIDEBOOK

This guidebook will help you to become a better problem solver. For some, these skills will be rather new. For others, it will be a matter of applying those skills that you already know to a different part of your life, such as applying certain decision-making strategies that you use all the time at work to problems you are experiencing with relationships. In any case, this guidebook is specifically geared to help you cope more effectively with stressful problems in order to improve your overall quality of life. Remember, this program is based on decades of scientific clinical research—that is very important to us. We do not wish to offer advice that we *think* might be helpful—rather, we wish to present guidelines that have been shown, time after time, study after study, to be effective in helping people of all ages to cope more effectively with life's stresses and to impact positively on their well-being.

In the next chapter, we provide an overview of the five steps to becoming an effective problem solver. This is followed by a self-test in Chapter 3 geared to help you obtain a better understanding of your current problem-solving strengths and limitations. We offer this test in order to determine where in particular you might need help and where such aid may not be especially warranted. These will be followed by chapters that provide specific and detailed training in each of the five steps of our model. Finally, we provide examples of how to apply this model to various common life problems.

## SOME IMPORTANT POINTS TO REMEMBER

- *Write things down.* It is a good idea for you to buy a notebook or journal, as there will be times when you need to write things down. Throughout this guide we describe how to use various

problem-solving worksheets that can help improve your ability
to use the various problem-solving tools.

- *Practice, practice, practice.* Similar to any skill, such as driving,
playing a sport, or learning a musical instrument, improvement
only comes with persistent practice. Take for example learning
how to play golf or tennis. It would be silly to think that all you
needed to do was read a book quickly and practice only occasionally. If you truly wanted to become a decent tennis player,
it is likely that you would want to practice as many times as
possible. Sometimes it is a matter of practicing your backhand
swing over and over again, and sometimes it involves playing
entire matches with someone slightly better than you. In the
same way, in order for any of these skills to be helpful, you need
to *practice!* We know that at various times it becomes very difficult to persist, especially when progress is slow. However, if
your initial attitude is one of accepting that changing your life
will take practice and persistence, rather than hoping that this
is the "magic pill," it is more likely that you will be ultimately
successful. Remember—this is for you and you are worth it.
Change takes time—"Rome wasn't built in a day"—neither can
you expect yourself to change overnight.

- *Be an active reader.* Read this book more slowly than you might
a novel. Stop when you have a question and take the time to
really think about what is being said. Don't skip over parts of a
chapter in order to see how it ends. Think about different situations in your life where a particular idea can be useful. Think
about how you might need to change the strategy slightly to
adapt to a different situation. Think about how you might share
your experiences with your spouse, friends, or family members.
Finally, it is likely that the more you re-read sections that are
relevant to you, the more that you will learn and be able to ultimately change.

- *Track your progress.* Be sure to complete the worksheets where
we ask you to rate your progress. That way, you can determine
how you are actually doing. In addition, keeping track of your
overall emotional well-being is also important. To do that, construct a simple scale that is relevant for you. For example, if
you have been feeling sad because of various relationship problems, use a scale from *1* (not at all sad) to *7* (very sad) to track
your progress as you attempt to cope with some of these difficulties. Rate your feelings at various intervals that are meaningful
for you (for example, every four weeks). Keep such records in
your notebook or journal. See if your level of sadness actually

decreases as you solve some of your stressful problems. Also, in Chapter 3, we provide a test of your overall problem-solving strengths and weaknesses. Another way to track your progress is to take this test when you read Chapter 3, but also again a few months later, after you have had a chance to learn and practice the five problem-solving steps described in this book as a means of evaluating your progress in improving your overall problem-solving ability.

- *Reward yourself.* Reinforce or reward yourself for trying to use these problem-solving skills. Also, reward yourself for making progress. Small changes are very important. Don't wait until you achieve your ultimate goal(s). A big victory is usually made up of a group of smaller ones. You can reward yourself by buying a new CD, going to the movies, getting tickets to a sports event, buying a new dress, going to a fancy restaurant, or doing something else that pleases you. Make the reward equal to the progress—for a lot of success, give yourself a *big* reward! Make sure that you associate the reward with your effort and progress.

# CHAPTER 2

# ADAPT: Five Steps to Solving Life's Problems

We cannot direct the wind, but we can adjust the sails.
                                    —*Dolly Parton*

### A WAY TO REMEMBER THE STEPS: *ADAPT*

We know that it is easier to remember a series of steps if you have an acronym to help recall what to do, especially when you are experiencing a strong emotion or difficult problem. In order to help you remember the five steps of effective problem solving, we will use the acronym *ADAPT*. We think this acronym highlights the notion that through problem solving, you can adapt or adjust more successfully to life's stresses and strains. As the Dolly Parton quote suggests, sometimes dealing with life requires us to adjust and adapt, as we are unable to control the world and everyone in it, no matter how much we would like to.

Each of these five steps has been shown, through scientific studies, to independently contribute to successful problem solving and can help you cope more effectively with the various stressful events that you encounter in life. We will devote a full chapter to each step later in this guidebook.

The five steps to effective problem solving include:

A = <u>A</u>*ttitude*. This step suggests that before you attempt to solve a problem, you should adopt a positive, optimistic *attitude* toward the problem and your own ability to cope with it.

D = <u>D</u>*efine*. After adopting a positive attitude, the next step involves correctly *defining* the problem by getting all the facts, identifying the obstacles to solving the problem, and specifying a realistic goal.

A = <u>A</u>*lternatives*. After coming up with a well-defined problem, you should then generate a variety of different *alternatives* for overcoming the obstacles and achieving your goal.

P = _P_redict. After generating a list of alternatives, you should *predict* the kind of consequences, both positive and negative, that might occur for each of these alternatives and choose the one that has the best chance of achieving your goal while minimizing costs and maximizing benefits.

T = _T_ry Out. When you have developed an action plan, *try out* the solution in real life and see if it works. If you are satisfied with the result, you have solved your problem. If you are not satisfied, then go back to "**A**" and *try again* to find a better solution.

These steps sound simple enough, right? Saying them is pretty simple, but actually putting them into practice with difficult problems involves a little more work. Sometimes it involves circling back through the previous steps if you are working on a complicated problem or having particularly strong emotional reactions to it. It is important to remember that large numbers of scientific studies indicate that this approach is an effective way to reduce stress, work through and decrease negative emotions, increase one's ability to adapt effectively to stressors, and improve one's overall quality of life. Before we describe each step, we suggest that you take a test to help you "diagnose" or assess your problem-solving strengths and limitations.

# CHAPTER 3

# Knowing Your Problem-Solving Strengths and Limitations

Knowledge itself is power.

*—Sir Francis Bacon*

## WHY EVALUATE YOUR PROBLEM-SOLVING ABILITIES, ATTITUDES, AND BELIEFS?

In order to become an effective problem solver, it's a good idea to first get a handle on your overall problem-solving abilities and attitudes. This can help you identify your own particular problem-solving strengths and weaknesses. In doing so, you can determine which skills you need only a little help with and which ones require extra training and practice.

In the next section, in order to help you better evaluate your general problem-solving abilities and skills, you will be asked to complete the *Problem-Solving Test.* This is a self-help test that is based upon a larger self-report questionnaire called the *Social Problem-Solving Inventory-Revised©* developed by psychologists Tom D'Zurilla, Art Nezu, and Albert Maydeu-Olivares. Based on research as to what real-life problem solving involves, these questions will allow you to assess your current problem-solving strengths, as well as specific areas that you will need to practice.

## HOW TO TEST YOUR PROBLEM-SOLVING STRENGTHS AND LIMITATIONS

### Instructions

To help you with your self-assessment, we provide the *Problem-Solving Test* for you to complete. Although the test will give you an idea of your problem-solving strengths and limitations, the most important part of

## PROBLEM-SOLVING TEST

1 = *Not at all true of me*
2 = *Somewhat true of me*
3 = *Moderately true of me*
4 = *True of me*
5 = *Very true of me*

1. I feel afraid when I have an important problem to solve.
2. When making decisions, I think carefully about my many options.
3. I get nervous and unsure of myself when I have to make an important decision.
4. When my first efforts to solve a problem fail, I give up quickly, because finding a solution is too difficult.
5. Sometimes even difficult problems can have a way of moving my life forward in positive ways.
6. If I avoid problems, they will generally take care of themselves.
7. When I am unsuccessful at solving a problem, I get very frustrated.
8. If I work at it, I can learn to solve difficult problems effectively.
9. When faced with a problem, before deciding what to do, I carefully try to understand why it is a problem by sorting it out, breaking it down, and defining it.
10. I try to do anything I can in order to avoid problems in my life.
11. Difficult problems make me very emotional.
12. When I have a decision to make, I take the time to try and predict the positive and negative consequences of each possible option before I act.
13. When I am trying to solve a problem, I often rely on instinct with the first good idea that comes to mind.
14. When I am upset, I just want to run away and be left alone.
15. I can make important decisions on my own.
16. I frequently react before I have all the facts about a problem.
17. After coming up with an idea of how to solve a problem, I work out a plan to carry it out successfully.
18. I am very creative about coming up with ideas when solving problems.
19. I spend more time worrying about problems than actually solving them.
20. My goal for solving problems is to stop negative feelings as quickly as I can.

21. I try to avoid any trouble with others in order to keep problems to a minimum.
22. When someone upsets me or hurts my feelings, I always react the same way.
23. When I am trying to figure out a problem, it helps me to stick to the facts of the situation.
24. In my opinion, being systematic and planful with personal problems seems too cold or "business-like."
25. I understand that emotions, even bad ones, can actually be helpful to my efforts at problem solving.

taking the test is to focus your attention on where you need the most practice. In this way, you can consider this guidebook as a type of personal trainer to help you "bulk up" and strengthen your psychological and emotional condition. In this test are statements regarding some ways that you might think, feel, and act when faced with problems in everyday living. Before beginning, take a few moments to think about something important in your life that bothers you a lot, but you don't immediately know how to make it better or stop it from bothering you so much. Such a problem could be something about yourself (such as your thoughts, feelings, behavior, health, or appearance), your interactions with other people (such as your family, friends, teachers, or boss), or your personal property and resources (such as your house, car, property, or money).

Please get out your notebook or journal now in order to write down your answers to the 25 questions. Please read each statement carefully and choose one of the numbers (that is, 1 through 5) on the 5-point scale included on the test that best describes how much that statement is true of you with regard to the way you face problems. See yourself as you *usually* think, feel, and act when you are faced with important problems in your life *these days.*

Write down the number in your notebook that best represents how you are. Answer all questions as honestly as possible (only you will know the results). Remember to answer how you truly are, *not* how you think you *should* be or would *like* to be. Also note the date in your journal when you are taking this test. After you learn and practice the five steps to effective problem solving, you may wish to re-take this test sometime in the future to determine your progress in improving your overall problem-solving abilities.

After you take this test, continue reading. But before we show you how to score this test, we provide a brief explanation of the major problem-solving dimensions that this test evaluates and corresponding examples of how both strengths and weaknesses in these areas occur in real life.

## MAJOR PROBLEM-SOLVING DIMENSIONS

Based on decades of clinical research, the following five dimensions of real-life problem solving have been identified:

- Positive problem orientation
- Negative problem orientation
- Rational problem-solving style
- Impulsivity/carelessness style
- Avoidance style

## PROBLEM ORIENTATION: YOUR PROBLEM-SOLVING ATTITUDE

*Problem orientation* refers to the manner in which we think and feel about problems in general, as well as about our ability to successfully cope with them. It is the "set of eyeglasses" that we constantly wear in viewing the world, especially with regard to problems in living. These thoughts and feelings can have a significant impact on our subsequent problem-solving efforts, as well as on our emotional and physical well-being. Research has identified two different types of problem-solving orientations, one being positive and the other negative.

### Positive Problem Orientation

A *positive orientation,* which is associated with more successful problem solving, involves a general set of attitudes to (a) view a problem as a challenge rather than a threat, (b) be realistically optimistic and believe that problems are solvable, (c) have the self-confidence to believe in one's ability to be a successful problem solver, (d) understand that solving difficult problems often takes persistence and effort, and (e) commit oneself to solve the problem rather than avoid it.

*Real-Life Example*

Sara had a very positive problem-solving orientation. After she broke her ankle while training for a professional golf match, she was faced with a painful rehabilitation, loss of income, and worries that the situation created added burden to her family. However, it was a help to her problem-solving efforts that she considered both the rehabilitation process and need to meet household expenses as *challenges* to face, rather than as overwhelming threats to her self-esteem or family. She was hopeful that her ability to be creative and the support she received from others would help her to improve the situation, even if it meant that there was no 100% perfect solution. She was confident that through persistence and effort, she could improve the situation in some ways.

## Negative Problem Orientation

A *negative orientation,* which is associated with unsuccessful problem solving, involves the general tendency to (a) view a problem as being a major threat to one's well-being, (b) doubt one's personal ability to solve a problem successfully, and (c) generally become frustrated, upset, and overcome with emotional distress when confronted with problems in living.

### Real-Life Example

Judy had a negative problem orientation. When she had an accident that was similar to the one described for Sara, she became fearful that the accident signaled the end of her ability to engage in physical activities in the same way as before, and that she would become a burden to her family (she was a homemaker and avid runner). This made it even more difficult for her family to help her to adjust to this set of problems, because she became very emotional whenever her husband tried to discuss any of the difficulties they were facing. She stated that such problems were proof that she was a burden to him. Moreover, she viewed her reduced access to exercise and need to have help cleaning the house as threats to her happiness, well-being, and self-esteem.

## PROBLEM-SOLVING STYLE

A problem-solving style refers to the general manner in which we react or respond to stressful problems. Research has identified three differing styles—one being adaptive and associated with successful problem solving (that is, rational problem-solving style), whereas the remaining two are related to unsuccessful problem solving and maladaptive outcomes (that is, impulsivity/carelessness style and avoidance style).

## Rational Problem Solving

This general style reflects an approach to solving problems that is planful, deliberate, and systematic. People who have strong rational problem-solving skills follow a type of "scientific method" when facing a problem and think in ways that most of us associate with careful and reasoned judgment. Such individuals tend to be those who gather facts and information about a problem, correctly identify the obstacles, set a realistic problem-solving goal, generate a variety of alternative options for overcoming the obstacles, identify and compare the pros and cons of these various alternatives, devise an effective solution plan based on this cost-benefit analysis, and carry the plan out optimally while carefully monitoring and evaluating the actual outcome.

### Real-Life Example

Bob, a divorced father of two, was someone who had strong rational problem-solving skills. When he was faced with the difficult problem of job relocation that required him moving further away from his kids, he first listed a series of goals that were important for him. He was specific and accurate in identifying obstacles, such as the cost of traveling to see his children, and he was creative in brainstorming possible alternative strategies to help meet his goals. He was careful not to make unfair assumptions about the reactions of his former wife, and he tried to get as many facts as possible to outline his situation. He weighed his decisions with an eye on both long- and short-term consequences not only for himself, but everyone involved, especially his kids. He ultimately was able to make some effective decisions and maintain his parenting role.

## Impulsivity/Carelessness Style

This problem-solving pattern is characterized by active attempts to solve a problem, but in a manner that tends to be careless, hurried, incomplete, and narrow. Such individuals consider only a few solutions to a problem, often impulsively going with the first idea that comes to mind. In addition, they overlook the range of possible consequences and inadequately monitor the outcome. Because of their impulsivity and carelessness, individuals high on this dimension are usually ineffective in problem-solving situations, often because they might say to themselves that it is a "good idea to go with one's gut feeling."

*Real-Life Example*

When Sondra's therapist asked her what led her to make certain choices, she would frequently say, "I don't know, I just wanted to ... isn't that ok?" For Sondra, it clearly was not. Without thinking through various situations and what made them a problem for her, or developing realistic goals, she often found herself acting on impulses to give herself an emotional lift, like engaging in e-mail gossip with a friend or drinking heavily without considering the consequences and disappointments that often followed her decisions. Her impulsivity usually was geared to make her feel better immediately, rather than to attempt to solve the real problem.

## Avoidance Style

This second maladaptive problem-solving style is characterized by tendencies to procrastinate, be passive, deny the existence of problems, and depend on others to resolve one's difficulties. Persons high on this dimension are more likely to avoid problems rather than confront them head on, put off problems for as long as possible, wait for problems to resolve themselves rather than attempt to solve them, and try to shift responsibility for solving their problems to others. Because of their tendencies to avoid or deny problems, such individuals are generally ineffective in coping with stressful difficulties.

*Real-Life Example*

People were often frustrated with Jake. He was a friendly guy who often made promises that he couldn't keep, such as inviting friends to his house without checking on other family plans, or volunteering to buy something for one of his kids without considering the consequences to the family budget. Jake came from a rigidly structured home where he never had the opportunity to do what he wanted. He hated having to think about money, or getting permission from other people to do something he wanted to do. Unfortunately, his avoidance of any planning or willingness to take time to realistically consider the consequences of his decisions led to a pattern of disappointing others by having to take back his promises.

## INSTRUCTIONS FOR SCORING YOUR TEST

Now that you know what makes up effective and ineffective problem solving, let's determine your personal problem-solving strengths and limitations. Below are specific instructions on how to both score and interpret the test.

## What Are Your General Problem-Solving Strengths and Weaknesses?

You can obtain your scores by adding together the numbers you listed for each of the five problem-solving scales listed next. These scales are divided into problem-solving strengths and problem-solving limitations. It is helpful to think of problem-solving ability in much the same way that you think about physical exercise and training. In a way, increasing your problem-solving strengths and reducing your problem-solving weaknesses helps to get you "in psychological shape" to manage the life problems that we all face on a day-to-day basis and to maintain your mental, emotional, and physical health.

### Scales of Problem-Solving Strengths

Your *Positive Attitude* score: add scores for items 5 + 8 + 15 + 23 + 25
Total Positive Attitude score (1): _____
Your *Rational Problem-Solving Skills* score: 2 + 9 + 12 + 17 + 18
Total Rational Problem-Solving Skills score (2): _____

### Explanation of Scores

For both the *Positive Attitude* scale and the *Rational Problem-Solving Skills* scale, scores below 12 indicate that you are in need of education (through carefully reading this book in a step-by-step method), training, and practice (either on your own or with your counselor's help if you are seeing someone in treatment) in order to "build up your problem-solving muscles" and improve your psychological resilience for the stress of daily problems.

Scores between 12 and 18 indicate that you have some strengths but can probably benefit from practicing to improve your rational problem-solving skills, positive attitude, or both.

Scores of 18 to 25 indicate that you already have positive attitudes and/or strong rational problem-solving skills. This is likely to enhance your practice with other problem-solving areas and make learning other problem-solving skills much easier because you are already in good psychological condition or shape.

### Scales of Problem-Solving Weaknesses

Your *Negative Attitude* score: add scores for items 1 + 3 + 7 + 11 + 16
Total Negative Attitude score (3): _____

Your *Impulsivity/Carelessness* score: add scores for items 4 + 13 + 20 + 22 + 24

Total Impulsivity/Carelessness score (4): \_\_\_\_\_

Your *Avoidance* score: add scores for items 6 + 10 + 14 + 19 + 21

Total Avoidance score (5): \_\_\_\_\_

For all of these scales, the scores indicate an opposite direction than the scales for (1) and (2). Scores above 12 indicate that you have some characteristic ways of dealing with problems that may get in the way of your problem-solving efforts.

A *Negative Attitude* score of 12 or higher indicates that you may have the tendency to think about problems in ways that are inaccurate and have difficulty managing the emotions that are often present when you are under stress. The higher the score, the more negative your problem-solving orientation, the more work will be required to change such negative thinking patterns.

An *Impulsivity/Carelessness* score of 12 or higher indicates that you may have the tendency not to "look before you leap" and may often make decisions that are not in your best interest. You will need to learn how to tolerate or reduce negative emotions and use your feelings to help you stop, think, define your problem, and consider different options *before* acting.

An *Avoidance* score of 12 or higher indicates that you have a tendency to avoid problems. This pattern of reacting to problems is of little to no help with the problem-solving process and often seriously impairs one's effectiveness in coping with challenging difficulties. You may find yourself withdrawing or leaving the room when engaged in an interpersonal argument, or pushing thoughts and feelings out of your head and distracting yourself when worried or sad. You probably need to work on reducing your fears or tolerating the anxiety you experience when facing problems.

## BEGINNING YOUR PROBLEM-SOLVING TRAINING (PST) WORKOUT

Having a better understanding of your problem-solving strengths and weaknesses, you are now ready to begin learning and practicing new skills in a way that will particularly benefit you and help you deal more effectively with stressful problems in general. In many ways, you will be strengthening your coping skills to more effectively manage life's problems, much in the way you might be strengthening your muscles if you were working out in a gym. As you go through this guide, particularly focus your attention on those areas of weaknesses that were identified by your scores on the *Problem-Solving Test*. It is also important to recognize any of the strengths that you already have and remain aware of how they can help you with your problem-solving efforts. Remember it is advisable that even if you have some significant strengths and require little additional help in other specific areas, it is still worthwhile to undergo all of the training in order to learn how your strengths in these areas can boost your overall problem-solving fitness as much as possible. You never know what you might learn, and it will be fun for you to flex your problem-solving muscles.

In general, the goals of this program, in order to help you become an effective problem solver, are to:

- Enhance your positive problem attitude
- Reduce your negative problem attitude
- Improve your rational problem-solving skills
- Reduce any tendencies to be impulsive or careless
- Reduce any tendencies to be avoidant

## REACTIONS TO A SPECIFIC PROBLEM

In addition to having a good understanding of your *general* problem-solving strengths and weaknesses, it is also important to learn how your thoughts, feelings, and actions in a given problem situation can help or hinder your success at solving that problem. For example, at times the way we *think* about a problem can greatly hinder ("This problem is way too hard to solve," "This is not really a problem," "I'm so bad with decisions") or enhance ("Even though this problem seems difficult, I will try my best") our success in solving it.

Moreover, how we *feel* ("This problem is complicated and scary" or "Even though this problem makes me worried, I feel confident I can solve it") about a problem can also affect our chances of being an effective problem solver. Which type of feeling or emotional reaction do you think makes it *less* difficult to solve the problem? Which type of feeling do you think makes it *more* difficult to cope with stress?

If certain thoughts or feelings in a given problem situation make it more difficult, then it is important to try to prevent them from making the problem even worse. Before we can do that, however, we must first learn to identify what we are actually thinking and what we are actually feeling in a given situation. To that end, we have developed a *Problem-Solving Worksheet* that is described below. Notice that the worksheet allows you to write down your thoughts, feelings, and actions regarding various problems that you encounter. We suggest that you get in the habit of writing down and describing the problems that you are experiencing in this format, your thoughts and feelings about the problem, as well as what you actually did to resolve or cope with it. In this way, you can begin to get a better picture of how your thoughts and feelings either help or hinder your problem-solving attempts.

Take out your notebook or journal once again in order to provide information in the following five areas of the *Problem-Solving Worksheet:*

1.  Briefly describe the problem.
2.  Describe your *thoughts*—before, during, and after the problem occurred.
3.  Describe your *feelings*—before, during, and after the problem occurred.
4.  Describe your *behavior*—what you actually did to try to cope with the problem.
5.  Rate how pleased you are with your coping attempts using a scale of 1 (not at all pleased) to 5 (very pleased).

Take a few moments right now to consider a problem that you recently faced. Perhaps it is a major difficulty or hardship, or a smaller annoying or frustrating hassle. See if you can identify what made this a problem for you, your thoughts and feelings about the problem, and what you did to try to solve the problem. Remember that thoughts and feelings are different. *Thoughts* refer to things you say to yourself like "What will I do now?," "They bug me and push my buttons," or "There's no way to solve this problem." *Feelings,* on the other hand, reflect what you are subjectively experiencing emotionally and can usually be summed up in one or two words (such as angry, scared, sad, lonely, elated, or numb). If you find yourself writing down your feelings with a statement such as "I felt as though he/she no longer cared for me," this represents more of a thought (that the person has changed their feelings toward you), and should be written down as a thought. A feeling involves how you would describe what it felt like when you told yourself this (for example, sad, angry, embarrassed, disappointed).

Try completing this *Problem-Solving Worksheet* several times. Take a careful look at what you wrote down. As you fill out the form for several problem situations, you may notice specific types of thoughts and feelings that occur or notice some patterns. When you are overwhelmed with negative feelings or repeat thought patterns that turn out to be inaccurate, exaggerated, or extra hard on yourself, these will be important patterns to change through the techniques you read about in this guidebook.

We know that you might be eager to begin learning and practicing the five steps to effective problem solving. But before we delve into these steps beginning with Chapter 4, we offer a set of three guidelines in the next section that can make the overall process of problem solving much easier for you. They can help you to become a better problem-solving multi-tasker.

Sherlock Holmes, the famous fictional detective who possessed great intelligence, would often characterize very difficult problems as a "three pipe problem," meaning that it would take smoking at least three pipes worth of tobacco before he would be able to solve the problem. Stressful real-life problems, in and of themselves, can be difficult to solve. But what makes it even more of a challenge is the limits on our ability to multi-task. This expression has become popular in the current computer age to describe the act of performing several tasks at the same time. Whereas a powerful computer can be a successful multi-tasker, due to the limited capacity of the human brain, this becomes difficult for us when attempting to solve real-life problems.

According to cognitive psychologist Marvin Levine, the conscious mind actually engages in three important activities during problem solving: (a) it takes in information from the environment (for example, inputs data); (b) "displays" that information when needed (that is, remembers or retrieves information from our memory banks); and (c) manipulates information that is remembered and attempts to comprehend it (that is, combines information, adds and subtracts information, tries to see how different pieces fit together).

However, according to Levine, the capacity of the conscious mind is limited in that it cannot perform all three activities efficiently at the same time, especially when the quantity and/or complexity of the information is substantial. Often, one activity interferes with another. For example, when we try to remember important information about a problem, this very act may, under certain conditions, interfere with our ability to comprehend other aspects of the problem.

Given this limited capacity (unfortunately we cannot go out to a computer store and buy more memory or power for our brains), what can we do when faced with a problem in life?

## Ways to Facilitate Problem-Solving Multitasking

Lucky for us, not only did Dr. Levine describe the problem of limited ability, but he also provided some simple ways to overcome such barriers (our guess is that he is a very effective problem solver!). Basically, he suggests using three rules that can be particularly useful for enhancing the process of problem solving. These include externalization, visualization, and simplification.

*Externalization* involves displaying information *externally* as often as possible. Simply put—write ideas down, draw diagrams to show relationships, make lists. This procedure relieves the conscious mind from having to actively display information being remembered, which allows one to concentrate more on other activities, such as creatively thinking of various solutions. Thus far, we have requested that you buy a notebook or journal in order to write things down. Many of the exercises in this book request that you make lists. Now you know why!

*Visualization* highlights the notion of using visual imagery whenever possible during the problem-solving process. To apply this rule, for example, you can use your imagination to visualize the problematic situation and rehearse solution alternatives. Research has demonstrated convincingly that visualization is a powerful tool that fosters our ability to remember, as well as to better comprehend information. Some of our problem-solving learning activities request you to use this rule. For example, in the next chapter, you will be provided with the opportunity to visualize certain problem-solving goals.

*Simplification* involves breaking down or simplifying problems in order to make them more manageable. To apply this rule, you should focus only on the most relevant information, break down complex problems into more manageable smaller problems, and translate complex, vague, and abstract concepts into more simple, specific, and concrete terms. This rule will also be recommended throughout this guidebook. One way to practice this rule at this point is to go back and look over one of your completed *Problem-Solving Worksheets*. Ask yourself the question—"If a friend read this information, would he or she understand it or did I use vague and ambiguous language and ideas?" If the answer is "no," go back and try to rewrite the information using the simplification rule. If that proves difficult, try to visualize talking to your friend to better determine what kinds of language you should use in order to really get your points across. Write this down, look over it, and try to simplify once again!

Now that you are armed with these three general rules to problem-solving multitasking, you are ready to begin learning and practicing the five steps to effective problem solving. We begin in Chapter 4 with helping you to enhance your problem-solving attitude.

# Step 1: Attitude: Enhancing Your Problem-Solving Capacity

## (Adapt)

In the middle of difficulty lies opportunity.

—*Albert Einstein*

The positive mind has greater solving power.

—*Alexander Cockhart*

### WHY SHOULD I ADOPT AN OPTIMISTIC ATTITUDE?

As we have indicated previously, a positive problem orientation can have a significant positive impact on how successful you are in solving problems and coping with stressful situations. Substantial research has demonstrated that a negative problem-solving attitude is associated with higher levels of depression, anxiety, anger, hopelessness, poor self-esteem, and pessimism. On the other hand, a strong positive attitude toward problem solving and problems in living is associated with more successful problem resolution, more hopefulness, and better emotional health. Therefore, it is important to try to be optimistic.

We are not suggesting that you believe that "life is a bowl of cherries!" Rather, we encourage you to adopt the belief that problems are a normal part of life and that if you extend effort and time, you will be able to adequately deal with most of them. A better phrase is "realistic optimism"—that is, not blindly thinking that everything will be okay, but that there are steps you can take to improve your problems so that everything is not *all* bad. Another way of looking at this is to think more that "the glass is half full, rather than the glass is half empty," while also realizing that you can develop skills that can add a little more water in the glass!

## OVERCOMING COMMON OBSTACLES TO ADOPTING A POSITIVE ORIENTATION

There are often certain obstacles that make it difficult for people to adopt a positive orientation. Such barriers include:

- Poor self-confidence
- Negative thinking
- Negative emotional reactions

If any or all of these barriers exist for you, the exercises contained in this chapter are provided to help you overcome them. What were your scores on the *Problem-Solving Test* specifically concerning the Positive and Negative Attitude scales? If you had a score on the Positive Attitude scale of less than 12 and/or a score of 12 or greater on the Negative Attitude scale, then you should spend additional time and effort working on skills presented in this chapter. If you are working with a therapist or counselor, it can be very helpful to ask their advice about which ones are important for you to particularly practice.

## OVERCOMING POOR SELF-CONFIDENCE: VISUALIZING SUCCESS

At times, one's lack of self-confidence or sense of hopelessness can result in an inability to see the light at the end of the tunnel. In other words, some people might say that they just can't see themselves successfully resolving a problem or achieving a particular goal. Sometimes it's hard to believe that anyone is able to handle a difficult and complex problem. However, research has shown that through *visualization,* people can learn to become more optimistic by visualizing a positive outcome.

Most people can learn to visualize. You visualize when you daydream, remember a past experience, picture a future vacation in your mind, or think of people that you know. Visualization is a powerful tool that can help us fulfill our dreams and achieve our life goals. In sports, it is very common for athletes to use visualization to help their speed, strength, or performance. For example, gymnasts and skaters are taught to visualize a routine they will perform at a competition; basketball players are taught to visualize the ball going into the hoop. Practicing visualization actually improves their performance.

With regard to the power of visualization to create hopefulness, one particularly profound story about visualization as a means of increasing optimism about a better future was described by Viktor Frankl, psychiatrist, author, and holocaust survivor. In his book, *Man's Search for*

_Meaning,_ Dr. Frankl describes a person's ability to visualize the future as "salvation in the most difficult moments of our existence." He recalls the poignant and powerful memories of his experience of pain and humiliation in a Nazi concentration camp and the endless problems that continually consumed him. He also described experiencing a type of personal epiphany, when during some of his darkest moments, he was able to force his mind and thoughts to another time and place. He described a visualization experience where he pictured himself standing at a podium in a warm and well-designed lecture room, with a full and attentive audience, giving a lecture on "the psychology of the concentration camp." He stated "[B]y this method I succeeded somehow in rising above the situation, above the sufferings of the moment, and I observed them as if they were already past ... emotion which is suffering, ceases to be suffering as soon as we form a clear picture of it" (p. 95). Those familiar with Dr. Frankl's biography know that after he survived the atrocities of this experience, he did go on to become an internationally known psychiatrist and author, who actually lived out his visualization to an extent that no one would have believed possible. We are not suggesting that simply visualizing a solution to difficult and complex problems alone will solve them. However, we are confident that people who can successfully visualize an improved future or a problem solved are more likely to be motivated to persevere in their problem-solving efforts.

The following visualization exercise asks you to use your imagination in order to "travel to the future" _after_ you successfully solved a difficult problem. Do _not_ think about how you got there—just that you did reach your problem-solving goals. Close your eyes and try to imagine where you are, who you are with, what you are thinking, and what you are feeling. Remember—it doesn't matter how you were able to solve the problem, just that a difficult problem was solved. Choose a problem that you are currently experiencing difficulty with—visualize being on the other side of the obstacles. How is your life different with this problem solved? How are you feeling? How are you feeling now as compared to before the problem was solved? Try to imagine _all_ of the positive consequences associated with having solved the problem. Try to see the light at the end of the tunnel.

At times, when people feel overwhelmed, they pay more attention to all the negative feelings associated with the problem, rather than the potential positive consequences associated with the problem being solved. This exercise is simply to help you to _experience_ something positive in order to feel at least a bit more motivated to try to do something. Give yourself some time alone to engage in this visualization exercise. Try your best to actually visualize yourself having solved a problem. It may be helpful to write down your reactions in your journal. Be sure to note the date.

If this exercise was not helpful at all, or if it was _particularly_ helpful, we have included a more extensive version of this exercise in the appendix.

It may not have been helpful for some because it sometimes is difficult to visualize by oneself. In the second exercise, we provide an actual script that can be tape-recorded in order to make visualization easier. On the other hand, for those who found this exercise helpful, a second one can only add to your ability to become a problem-solving expert.

## OVERCOMING NEGATIVE THINKING—LEARNING TO "THINK HEALTHY"

A second barrier to adopting a positive problem-solving attitude might be *negative thinking*. Sometimes that negative thinking comes to us in the form of rules. We all think according to rules that are in our heads. The problem is that some of these rules are not very accurate and are sometimes based on notions that we have learned to say to ourselves over a long period of time. Some thoughts that go through our heads are not even in our day-to-day awareness. For example, what would you say if we asked you if you thought that it was realistic or possible for someone to be loved by everyone 100% of the time? You would be correct in saying that, of course, this is not possible. Yet, every day, people allow themselves to *feel* badly and react with fear and surprise when they find out that someone does not like them. In such a case, they become sad or angry over something that is not possible to ever expect in the first place. They don't focus on the many who do care, but rather on that one person who doesn't. This can leave someone feeling like they are constantly failing or not meeting up to their own expectations.

However, when people use this problem-solving tool of healthy thinking, they can have a different outlook on life. Their happiness is much more in *their* control because they focus on what they are doing, trying, achieving, and experiencing, and *not* what other people expect or how other people react. In other words, they are following "healthy thinking rules" that are more accurate, objective, and rational. Many people have found these "rules" to be very helpful to decrease feelings of anxiety and depression, or when experiencing problems with other people, such as family members or co-workers. It can also be used as a preventative method for managing stress and promoting feelings of control and self-confidence.

## HEALTHY THINKING RULES

These are rules to live by because they will help you to gain perspective at times of stress—practicing *applying* these rules can help you to minimize emotional distress by helping you to think more realistically and objectively.

> Rule #1: How we think often affects the way we feel. How I feel about a situation is based on what I think about the situation.

Situations don't make you anxious, depressed, or angry. It's what you say to yourself about the situation that leads you to feel a certain way. If you choose to interpret or *think about* situations differently, you will *feel* different. As Marcus Aurelius, the Roman emperor, stated centuries ago—"Our life is what our thoughts make it." Even centuries before that, Buddha said something very similar—"With our thoughts we make the world."

We describe this as the *ABC Model of Thinking,* where A = the _a_ctivating event or situation (an event that you experience), B = the _b_elief (what you believe or say to yourself about the situation), and C = the emotional _c_onsequence (your emotional reaction based on your beliefs). For example, imagine that a coworker is not cooperative with an assignment that you asked him to complete. You can interpret the situation to mean many different things. For example, you might think that the co-worker has something against you, that he is lazy, that he believes your request to be foolish, that he didn't understand what you wanted him to do, that he had more respect for the previous person in your position than he has for you, that he is going through a very difficult personal crisis, *or* that he is afraid that his work won't be good enough so he's putting it off. Think about how each interpretation could result in very *different* emotions. Using healthy, rational thinking rules means that you focus on *facts* and stop making assumptions or having expectations about yourself or others that are unfair. In this example, even if your coworker's behavior is based upon negative feelings for you, this is a behavior that *he* or *she* (not you) must change.

> Rule #2: Nothing is 100% perfect—problems are a normal part of life—I can't control the whole world, no matter how hard I try.

The conditions for people or things to be otherwise just don't exist. To say things *should* be otherwise is to believe in magic. Situations (and people) are what they are because of a long series of events, some of which include interpretations, responses to the things we tell ourselves, and so on. Sad or bad things happen, and life is not fairly balanced for all—that's just the way it is, as disappointing as that sounds. Accepting this fact will keep you focused on the goals that you set for yourself and keep you going despite periodic setbacks. Remember—if you don't try, nothing will ever get better. But life isn't problem-free. We can expect problems to occur. Remember, as Dolly Parton stated—"You can't direct the wind, but you can adjust the sails!"

Rule #3: All humans make mistakes—even me.

This is an inescapable fact. If you do not set *reasonable* goals for yourself and others, or allow for periodic acts of stupidity, you greatly increase the chances of disappointment and unhappiness. However, if you *do* expect that you will make your fair share of mistakes and believe that these can actually become *learning* experiences, think of the possibilities for gaining new skills that you will have in the future! We all make mistakes. We can try hard not to make them—but we shouldn't punish ourselves when we do make a mistake. It's a good idea to give ourselves a break sometimes.

Rule #4: Every minute I spend thinking negative thoughts actually takes away from the pleasure of focusing on positive aspects of my life.

This rule highlights the personal choice we make to repeat and persevere with negative thoughts when there is often an equal amount of positive thoughts that are available. Yes, it's really a choice! Even when people are coping with a major loss, such as the death of loved one, positive thoughts or memories about the person or the relationship can be a focus of joy. It's up to us to choose which way we wish to think.

Rule #5: It takes two to have a bad relationship or conflict (also known as the 30% rule).

Before beginning a whole series of accusations or blame, or thinking of yourself as an innocent victim, remember that with few exceptions, any person involved in an argument is contributing at least 30% (if not more) to keeping it going. Even if you have been unfairly accused or treated (remember Rule #2 above), maybe there are things that you could do differently to prevent this from happening in the future. You don't have to take *all* of the blame, in order to be *part* of the solution.

Rule #6: Forget winning—learning lasts longer—I can think of problems as challenges, not as threats.

In contests where there is a winner, there is also a loser. Most people don't like to lose, so they get stuck on being the one who wins. The next time you face a difficult situation or conflict with someone, try saying to yourself, "Well, this is very challenging—it truly makes no difference if I win—after all, what would I win? More important, what is one thing I can learn from this situation?" Most often both people can learn important lessons, even if they don't win the argument or succeed in proving someone else wrong. When problems occur, it is beneficial to try to focus on what we can actually learn from the situation—we can gain new skills, learn how to prevent a similar problem from occurring in the future, or find out something about ourselves that is important to discover. _We can actually grow from adversity._ Think of what we can gain from our problems! As American poet Anne Bradstreet stated—"If we had no winter, the spring would not be so pleasant; if we did not sometimes taste of adversity, prosperity would not be so welcome."

## How to Apply These Rules

It is helpful to focus on one or two of these rules that are most helpful to you and say them frequently to yourself. For example, let's say that you have looked over the list and see that Rule #3 ("All humans make mistakes") really has meaning for your life. For example, you find yourself reacting with anger whenever someone gives you any kind of criticism (even constructive criticism) because you are so afraid to admit that you sometimes make mistakes. Don't wait for a situation to occur when your anger already has been triggered. Practice saying the rule to yourself many times throughout the day and even ask for advice or constructive criticism. Practice stating the rule in different ways to yourself. For example, in addition to "All humans make mistakes—even me," try making the rule more personal to yourself with different versions, such as "I _can_ make mistakes," "Good people _do_ make mistakes," "Recognizing my mistakes will help to _learn_ from them," or "It is irrational and foolish to expect that I am the only human being who _never_ makes mistakes." Then, try admitting a mistake to yourself for practice.

When you do find yourself feeling sad, anxious, angry, confused, or distressed, try to apply the _ABC Model of Thinking_ as described under Rule #1. Try to identify the "B," that is, what you are saying to yourself or believe about the event "A" that is making you feel distressed. If you find that you are using words such as should, must, ought, or have to (for example, "I _have to_ get that promotion," "She _should_ like me," "I _have to_ solve this problem ASAP"), then it is likely that you are engaging in _unhealthy_ thinking. Try to argue against such negative self-talk using some of the arguments presented in each of the _healthy thinking rules_ described above. In addition, question any "catastrophic words" (for example, "This is the worst thing that could happen," "I'll never be the same," "Life is over") that you are saying to yourself and try to assess the *real* consequences. Even severe accidents or medical illnesses do not automatically mean the end of life. Remember Viktor Frankl and his visualizations that helped him cope with being in a concentration camp.

One way to help combat negative self-talk is to be able to replace it with more realistically optimistic self-talk. For example, look over the list of Positive Self-Statements contained in Table 4.1. These are not statements that we simply thought of—rather, they were provided to us by individuals diagnosed with cancer who participated in many of our problem-solving programs for various medical patients. Several of these individuals actually wrote some of these statements down on 3" × 5" index cards and carried them in their wallets or purses in order to be able to take them out whenever they started to feel distressed. Others posted such a list on their refrigerators or bathroom mirrors during times of increased stress. Can you think of any to add to this list? Try to add to it and make a list in your journal or notebook.

### TABLE 4.1  Positive Self-Statements That You Can Use to Battle Your Negative Self-Talk

I can solve this problem!

I'm okay—feeling sad is normal under these circumstances.

I can't direct the wind, but I can adjust the sails.

I don't have to please everyone.

I can replace my fears with faith.

It's okay to please myself.

There will be an end to this difficulty.

If I try, I can do it!

I can get help from _____ if I need it.

It's easier, once I get started.

I just need to relax.

I can cope with this!

I can reduce my fears.

I just need to stay on track.

I can't let the worries creep in.

Prayer helps me.

I'm proud of myself!

I can hang in there!

## OVERCOMING NEGATIVE EMOTIONS: LEARNING TO USE YOUR NEGATIVE FEELINGS ADAPTIVELY

A third possible barrier to adopting a positive problem orientation is the experience of negative emotions. People experience upsetting feelings every day. However, emotions can be very tricky. Sometimes our feelings are a reaction to just one situation and they simply pass. At other times, we are bothered by upsetting feelings for longer periods of time. Problems like depression, anxiety, anger, and bereavement all involve distressful feelings. It is important for you to use this tool if you find that such feelings serve as an obstacle for you to adopt a positive orientation or if a strong emotional reaction hinders your ability to effectively resolve a particular problem.

It is very common for most people to need some help managing their negative feelings. Emotional problems are often the reason why people seek help from counselors. The following instructions are designed to give a step-by-step approach so you can use the power of feelings adaptively and to your advantage. By practicing these steps, you will be more aware of your negative feelings and be able to use them as signals or cues that a problem exists, rather than simply dwell on them, only to feel worse. In addition, this approach can help you deal better with such feelings, as well as with the problem that is causing your distress.

Consider the idea that negative emotions are one of nature's gifts to you. It is a mistake to view negative feelings as being all bad. How can that be true? Actually, negative emotions can be thought of as nature's way of telling you that something is wrong and that a problem exists. In this manner, they are helpful to our ultimate well-being, even though they may be unpleasant at the time. Follow these steps in order to learn how to use your feelings as cues.

*Step 1.* Throughout the day, any time when you begin to feel distressed or physically uncomfortable, stop to notice what you are feeling and how intense these feelings are. Try to put into words what emotion you notice first. Write them down in your notebook or journal.

*Step 2.* Now notice where you experience this feeling the most. Do you have physical sensations, like your heart pounding, a lump in your throat, or your face flushing? Do you say things to yourself, like "I can't take this," "I don't need this," "I hate to feel this way," "I'll show him what it feels like," or "I give up"? As you begin to get familiar with how you experience your own emotions, consider all of these signs (that is, both the physical sensations and things you say to yourself) as cues, signals, or clues that something is going on, something like a problem. *Then go immediately to Step 3.*

*Step 3. Stop and think.* Imagine a stop sign or a flashing red traffic light as a way to help you stop. This step means stopping all action, almost like you would when you press the pause button on your video player or movie camera. You are going to stop *all* actions (even talking) for a few seconds to become more aware of your emotions. In this frozen moment in time, allow yourself to experience the emotion and then identify what you are feeling. *Inhibit the tendency to try to feel better before realizing what is truly going on or to deny the feeling in order to make it go away.* Those of you who scored 12 or greater on the Avoidance scale of the *Problem-Solving Test* are likely to especially need to practice this step.

*Step 4.* This step is geared to help you learn to be wise—in other words, to be able to better understand what your emotions are trying to tell you. When you react only with your feelings, it is difficult to listen to the logical or rational part of your mind. In such a case, you are likely to act impulsively with more feelings. For example, in reaction to something that has happened, you might get angry. However, for some people, getting angry leads to embarrassment, then embarrassment leads to fear, then fear leads to more anger. In this manner, one might never get away from these bad feelings and the original reason why you became angry (which may be natural and predictable) is lost.

On the other hand, if you think only with logic (for example, like Dr. Spock for those of you who are Star Trek fans), you may disregard the important information that your emotions are telling you. For instance, suppose that you are feeling sad because you are lonely. Your rational thinking may lead you to discount or discredit your feelings, which may lead you to be unaware of the importance of seeking more support or friendship from others.

What happens when we bring emotions and thinking together? In general, it takes *both* types of processes to be wise—in other words, to be able to use your emotions to let you know what is really going on. This can be hard work, because it means taking the time to figure out what important information your feelings are providing you. With this new wisdom, however, you will be able to answer the question of what your emotions are telling you. Having this information allows you to decide what to do next.

*Step 5.* This next step helps you to answer the question—"What are my emotions telling me?" Remember why you have emotions in the first place—to give you information. Your body is set up to react with certain feelings for very good reasons. Look at Table 4.2. It contains the type of information you should be looking for when you are trying to identify what your feelings are saying to you. We have also provided a few common examples of what the information may reveal.

Some of the information that a feeling tells you may point to an actual situation that you need to do something about. It may also involve

**TABLE 4.2   Emotions and What They May Be Telling You**

| What You Are Feeling | What Your Feelings Might Be Telling You | What This Information Might Reveal About You |
| --- | --- | --- |
| Fear | You feel that threat or danger is nearby. | What are you afraid of? Physical harm, being laughed at, feeling inferior, being rejected, getting fired? |
| Anger | You are being blocked from getting something you want. | What do you want? To be successful, a relationship, an accomplishment, to be loved? |
| Sadness | You have lost something significant. | What have you lost? A friend, lover, or partner; your power, status, or role; losing what you like to do; your importance? |
| Embarrassment | You believe that others can see your imperfections, mistakes, or problems. | What do they see? Your intellectual weaknesses, your emotions, your faults? |
| Guilt | You are focusing on something you regret. | What do you regret? That you hurt others? Is someone else telling you that you hurt them? |

something that you are telling yourself or a situation that you are having difficulty accepting. Therefore, the information you receive from feelings can let you know what situation you need to focus on changing, self-statements that are irrational, exaggerated or incorrect, or new situations or challenges that you must realistically confront.

_Step 6._ In order to achieve emotional balance in your life, it is important to work toward changing things that you can, becoming more realistic and accepting of things that you _cannot_ change, and learning how to know the difference. This is where _true_ wisdom comes from—learning to actually listen to your emotions and then apply your logical thinking to decide what you need to do. In other words—_stop and think._ Stopping and thinking allows you to put the brakes on a potentially fast-moving train that is carrying negative emotions as baggage and to determine your next move. As noted Nobel Peace Prize winner Albert Schweitzer stated decades ago—"Think first, then do." In other words, thinking before doing, or "looking before you leap," is more likely to lead to better problem solving. Those of you who scored 12 or higher on the Impulsivity/Carelessness scale of the *Problem-Solving Test* will likely need to particularly practice this skill.

## What Happens If My Negative Emotions Are Too Strong?

Here are some tips to help you to better control (not *erase,* otherwise you would become a robot without feelings) any disruptive negative emotions:

- If your emotions point to a situation where negative *thinking* may be responsible for the negative *feelings* (for example, "I didn't get the raise because I am stupid!") and you have difficulty "stopping that train," practice the healthy thinking rules exercise more frequently in order to help you overcome such negative thinking.
- If you are feeling tense, anxious, and are having difficulty relaxing, we provide a stress management exercise in the appendix, called "Deep Breathing." Visualization exercises have also been found to be very helpful to reduce stress. Therefore, we include another visualization exercise in the appendix as well that allows you to "go to a safe place" in order to reduce tension and anxiety.
- As repeated throughout this guidebook, it is highly likely that the reason why you might be experiencing distress is related to the various problems you currently are experiencing. As such, one way to attempt to decrease these negative emotions is to try to persevere in solving your current stressful difficulties in spite of feeling upset. Resolving many of these problems will likely lead to a major decrease in distress.
- If these suggestions are not helpful after concerted attempts, and you continue to experience high levels of anxiety or depression, it is possible that you may wish to seek professional help from a counselor or psychologist.

## WHAT IS YOUR PROBLEM? RECOGNIZING PROBLEMS WHEN THEY OCCUR

A positive problem orientation also emphasizes the notion that problems in living are common and as such, we should be able to recognize and identify problems when they occur. Experiencing psychological, family, physical, relationship, or financial stressors is likely to change your life in many ways—some of which may have led to additional difficulties. Although some people find that their lives can change for the better in certain stressful situations (for example, when ill, they may appreciate their family and friends more than before), most stressful situations create new and challenging problems.

We are certainly not suggesting that you need to be super-vigilant about looking for problems; rather, when something is going wrong, you are able to recognize the situation as a problem and thus, are likely to want to do something about it. How can you tell when a problem is occurring?

- *Use your feelings as a cue that a problem exists.* This notion was described in detail previously. Instead of labeling one's negative feelings as the problem, you should think of these feelings as a signal that a problem exists and then observe what is going on in an attempt to recognize the *real* problem that is causing these feelings. Common emotional consequences of stressful problems are anxiety, uncertainty, depression, anger, dissatisfaction, disappointment, confusion, guilt, feelings of inadequacy, and feelings of helplessness. Note that *feelings* in this context not only refer to emotional states (e.g., "I feel sad"), but also to physical symptoms (e.g., "I feel like there are butterflies in my stomach," "My head hurts just thinking about this," "I feel so shaky and jittery").
- *Use your behavior as a signal that a problem exists.* It is possible that you have tried some old methods of dealing with a problem that do not seem to be working now. Think of these unsuccessful attempts as another type of signal that a problem exists. However, don't think of your unsuccessful actions as the problem, but think of such actions as a signal to seek out and identify the problematic situation.
- *Use certain thoughts as cues that a problem exists.* In addition to negative emotions or ineffective behavior, certain thoughts may be indicators that a problem exists. Thoughts such as "I *should* have gotten a perfect score on that test, now I'll never get into medical school," "The bills seem to be piling high this month, I'll just forget about them for now because they just make me upset," "I *should* ask Sally to marry me even though I'm not sure—it's my 'gut feeling' and I should go with that" are ones that should signal that a problem exists.
- *Use a problem checklist.* In Table 4.3 is a checklist of problems to use in order to help you better pinpoint your own specific problems. Psychologists have actually developed multiple types

of problem checklists to help their patients better identify some of their concerns. Remember that such checklists would not exist if *many* people did not experience problems. You are not alone! Millions of others may be experiencing similar types of difficulties at this very moment.

**TABLE 4.3   Common Problems Checklist**

---

*Psychological/Emotional Problems*
- ❑   Worries about the future
- ❑   Memory or concentration difficulties
- ❑   Feeling sad
- ❑   Feeling lonely
- ❑   Difficulty making decisions
- ❑   Getting angry at others

*Family Problems*
- ❑   Arguments with others
- ❑   Changing family roles
- ❑   Family expectations
- ❑   Family insensitivity
- ❑   Family responsibilities

*Medical Problems*
- ❑   Difficulties getting the right information
- ❑   Feel nervous to ask questions of my doctor
- ❑   Problems with medication
- ❑   Diet or lifestyle changes
- ❑   Feeling out of control

*Sexual Problems*
- ❑   Lost interest in sex
- ❑   Sexual difficulties or dysfunction
- ❑   Loss of availability of sex
- ❑   Guilt over sex

*Work-Related Problems*
- ❑   Work dissatisfaction
- ❑   Work pressures
- ❑   Problems with coworkers
- ❑   Financial problems
- ❑   Lack of recognition
- ❑   Insufficient funds for daily needs
- ❑   Lack of benefits
- ❑   Embarrassment over finances
- ❑   Unable to obtain work

---

*(continued)*

**TABLE 4.3    Common Problems Checklist** *(continued)*

*Legal Problems*

❏    Being sued
❏    Too many traffic tickets
❏    Income tax difficulties
❏    Custody battles

*Community Problems*

❏    Neighborhood is changing for the worse
❏    Unwanted construction
❏    Too close to noisy roads
❏    Property taxes too high
❏    Trash build-up
❏    Neighbors are too loud

## What Kinds of Problems Have You Been Experiencing?

Look over Table 4.3. This includes a brief list of problems in various categories that are common ones experienced by others. Review the list and note how many currently apply (or do not apply) to you right now. What kinds of problems are you experiencing? Are you experiencing any of the ones listed in the table? Are there any other problems? In your journal or notebook, list those problems that you are currently experiencing and would like to address. List them according to your priorities. Try to be as specific as possible. For example, one person we worked with was feeling lonely. Rather than just writing down that he felt lonely, he said, "Feeling lonely makes me feel angry and hopeless and then I'm not motivated to try to do things that I would otherwise probably enjoy."

Look over this list and try to identify a problem that you would like to work on right now. Put a star (*) or other notation next to it to highlight it. In the next several chapters of this guidebook, you will learn the remaining four steps to becoming an effective problem solver in order to successfully cope better with this problem as well as with others. As you improve the problems you are experiencing, you will also be reducing the obstacles to achieving some of the goals you set for yourself when you were visualizing the future. In the next chapter, we will move on to Step 2—defining a problem and setting realistic goals.

# CHAPTER 5

# Step 2: Defining Your Problem and Setting Realistic Goals

## (aDapt)

It isn't that they can't see the solution.
It's that they can't see the problem.

—*G. K. Chesterson*

## DEFINING THE PROBLEM

There is an old saying by John Dewey—"A problem well-defined is a problem half-solved." A similar adage is "Measure twice, cut once." Both sayings suggest the notion that if we take the time to fully understand the nature of the problem we are experiencing, solving it will take less time and effort. More importantly, paraphrasing Chesterton above, "seeing the problem" helps to "see the solution."

Defining a problem is similar to laying out a course or route to travel. Even if several people have the same destination, they may not all have the same resources, such as time or money, to be able to take the same exact trip. If one has never traveled to a particular destination, it becomes especially difficult due to its unfamiliarity. Simply looking at a map without knowing a specific destination would be overwhelming. As such, defining a problem is similar to first identifying on a road map where you wish to go. Another way of saying this is to first identify your goals. In this way, you can later determine how to get there (that is, your solution plan).

Correctly defining a problem involves the following five steps as described below:

- Seeking the available facts
- Describing the facts in clear language

- Separating facts from assumptions
- Setting realistic goals
- Identifying the obstacles to overcome

## SEEKING THE AVAILABLE FACTS

Sometimes people try to solve a problem before they know all the facts. It is likely that before you agree to buy a certain car, you wish to know all about it—how much gas mileage it gets, its safety record, what other consumers think about it, and so forth (at least you should!). Why do anything different with a personal problem? With any situation that is causing you distress, it is important to seek out any facts or information that are not readily available. If we don't actually know what the problem is, we might wind up working on the wrong one!

For example, one patient we worked with, Sam, was getting more and more angry because he felt that since he had been divorced, he experienced his family and friends as being overly worried and treating him very "delicately." This often led Sam to believe that they were avoiding him. He told us that they seemed very careful not to talk about his ex-wife and were starting to avoid telling him about good times they had for fear they would upset him. Sam thought that his friend Bill, particularly, was beginning to think of him as a "fragile person." This made Sam angry, which often led to arguments that left them both feeling sad and frustrated. However, after encouraging Sam to find out more about why his friend acted this way, he learned that Bill was starting to feel like there was nothing he could do to help Sam get past his divorce, and his avoidance had more to do with his own feelings of failure as a friend. Thinking of all the times Sam helped him made Bill feel like he was failing as a friend because he could not be of more help. Ironically, all Sam wanted from Bill was to behave toward him the way he always had and not try to make things better. As such, it seemed that one thing both Sam and Bill needed to do was to seek the available facts.

Sam was directed to learn to think of himself as a detective, scientist, or newspaper reporter, whose job was to get the facts. He was told to ask questions such as *who, what, when, where, why,* and *how.* He was further reminded that as a detective, if he were to "report back to headquarters," such questions would have to be answered in a manner that was objective and thorough in order to allow an uninformed person to understand what actually happened. You may have noticed that when talking to a counselor or therapist, these are the types of objective questions that they ask. Therefore, by learning to think like a detective or a news reporter when considering your own personal problems, you will be learning to serve as your own therapist.

How can you use this step to help you get the facts? Remember the externalization principle—write information down. Write down answers to the following questions in your notebook or journal regarding a current problem. This may be the problem you prioritized at the end of Chapter 5. On the other hand, it might be a different one. Read your answers—do you have *enough* facts? Do you need to get some more? Put on the "detective hat" and go out and seek some more facts if necessary. Add them to your list of facts about this problem.

- Who is involved?
- What happened (or did not happen) that bothers you?
- Where did it happen?
- When did it happen?
- Why did it happen? (i.e., known causes or reasons for the problem)
- How did you respond to the situation? (i.e., actions, thoughts, and feelings)

Sometimes it is difficult to try to sort out what is relevant or useful information when attempting to answer these types of questions. If you are experiencing this difficulty, remember the second multi-tasking principle—visualization! You can use the following visualization technique to help you identify relevant information in order to answer the above types of questions:

Close your eyes and reconstruct in your imagination a recent experience that was an instance of a recurring problem or part of a current, ongoing problem. First, imagine that you are in the situation (not viewing it as an observer) and experience it in your imagination as it actually happened. As you are experiencing the situation, ask yourself—"What am I thinking and feeling?" Next, repeat the experience, but this time as an observer, as if watching a movie or videotape of the situation. Play it in *slow* motion and ask yourself—"What is happening? What is the other person(s) saying, doing, and feeling? What am I saying, doing, and feeling?"

## DESCRIBING THE FACTS IN CLEAR LANGUAGE

Especially when we feel stressed, we tend to use language that is unclear. For example, Sam originally came to us stating that he felt that Bill was treating him "like he was some kind of psycho" and that he was making him feel so frustrated that "his head was going to explode." Being presented with these problems, imagine Sam's reaction if we told him that, based on such descriptions, we would get him a room on the psych ward and remove the fuse from his head so it wouldn't explode. Of course Sam's initial description provides a colorful way of explaining his feelings, but for us to help him, it became very important for Sam to be able to describe his feelings and problems using *clear* language. This is very much in keeping with the third problem-solving multitasking principle—*simplification*.

Another example involves a different patient we know, Jane, who came to us because of feelings of anxiety. She initially stated—"Riding in elevators is a nightmare. It's like I'm going to die or something!" A more accurate and factual description would be—"My anxiety is at its most intense when I ride in elevators. As the doors open and I step inside, my heart beats fast, my skin feels clammy, I think about my family's history of heart disease and have thoughts about dying. As soon as I step off, I have immediate thoughts of relief and feel my heart rate return to normal."

When we don't use clear language, we can blow things out of proportion or have other people misunderstand what we are saying. Reporters and detectives need to use clear language as well. For example, Sam, when angry, tended to overstate the frequency of his friend's avoidance. When he first described the situation, he indicated that his friend "never shared anything with him anymore." In fact, after being encouraged to focus on the facts and use clear language, he admitted that it happens only about half of the time that he originally claimed. This was a big difference.

## SEPARATING FACTS FROM ASSUMPTIONS

Sometimes people make assumptions, especially when they are emotional, without paying attention to this automatic thought process. Assumptions have a way of becoming facts before anyone tries to determine if they are really true. Continuing with the theme of thinking like a news reporter or a scientist, remember that such individuals are on the lookout for *objective* facts. A *fact* is something that most people would agree to be true; an *assumption* involves a person's *beliefs, opinions,* or *interpretations* without determining its validity.

If we act only on assumptions, we are likely to be unsuccessful in our problem-solving attempts. Therefore, we need to *separate facts from assumptions* before we act on unverified information. For example, getting back to Sam, he assumed that his friend, when he avoided telling him about positive things in his life, thought he was no longer any fun to be with and thought Sam was a burden. It was bad enough that this was not true (that is, an assumption), but he tended to blow this idea up even more and began to feel that Bill no longer valued him as a friend. Based on these supposed facts, Sam felt justified in his anger and his arguments. Further, his immediate reactions to such assumptions, and not actual facts, led to his continued anger, frustration, arguments, and sadness. So, in this case, Sam interpreted his friend Bill's change in behavior as evidence that he no longer wanted Sam for a friend, when the facts later revealed that Bill was fearful that he wasn't being as helpful as Sam needed him to be.

We have found that a useful exercise to help people to separate facts from assumptions is to show them pictures cut out from various magazines. The instructions would be to look at the picture for a few moments, put it down, and then begin writing everything they can think of to describe the picture. After writing down what they saw or thought was going on in the picture, the instructions are to look through the list and identify the things that they wrote that are absolute _facts,_ and only facts. Anything that is not a fact suggests that the person had an idea, opinion, or belief about the picture but was unsure as to whether it was true or not. This is identified as a belief, opinion, or assumption, for which one would need _more_ information to determine its validity.

You might find this exercise helpful or fun. Get some magazines, look for pictures that might be a bit ambiguous, and do the same— that is, look at it for a few moments, put it down, and write in your journal or notebook everything that you saw or think is going on in the photo. Now, have a friend or family member do the same. After both of you finish the task, look at each other's lists and see how much you agree. Do you have a tendency to assume too much? Are most of your observations actually facts? Do you tend to hold beliefs, opinions, or assumptions about what is going on without having all the facts? If you are seeing a counselor or therapist, this might be an exercise that you wish to do with him or her during one of your sessions. If you belong to a support group, it can be a useful group exercise to stimulate discussion about becoming more accurate in defining problems.

Now go back to your journal or notes where you described various facts about one of the problems that you are currently experiencing. Look over the facts. Did you use clear language, or words that make it difficult for someone else to really understand? Can you identify which facts are really assumptions? If so, you may need to put on the detective's hat and seek out additional facts to see if the assumption is really true or just an assumption. Be sure to use the questions that such individuals might use (_who, what, when, where, why,_ and _how_).

## Common Thinking Mistakes That Lead to False Assumptions

If you find the above exercise a bit difficult, and you continue to wonder if something is a fact or an assumption, the following is a list of questions that can help you even further. Research has identified several common thinking mistakes that are likely to result in false assumptions when one attempts to define a problem. Making such mistakes can lead to an incorrect problem definition. To help identify these mistakes, and especially to help you correct them, we suggest that you ask yourself the following questions when you are in doubt:

1. *Am I making an assumption without having enough facts to support it or rule out alternative interpretations?* People often make assumptions or inferences about other people's thoughts, feelings, intentions, or motives in certain situations. Because we are not mind readers, these assumptions are often incorrect. For example, when Jennifer turns down Frank's request for a date, he *incorrectly* concludes that she thinks he is a loser. To avoid making this mistake, you need to obtain enough facts to support your assumptions or to rule out alternative interpretations.

2. *Am I focusing only on some facts while ignoring other important ones?* People often focus only on certain selected facts and draw a conclusion based solely on this information while ignoring other important facts that actually contradict such a conclusion or support a very different one. For example, because John made an error in a baseball game and ignored the fact that several other players made more serious errors, he *incorrectly* concluded that he alone cost his team a victory. To avoid this mistake, you should always consider *all* the facts when drawing conclusions.

3. *Am I overgeneralizing?* Individuals often make *incorrect* assumptions about the general characteristics of people or situations on the basis of a single (and often trivial) event. For example, Sally fails the first exam in a course and concludes that she is a failure. Bill is rejected by Lisa when he asks for a date and assumes that *all* girls will reject him. Henry lies to Mary and she concludes that *all* men are liars and cannot be trusted. To avoid this type of thinking mistake, focus only on the situation at hand—don't overgeneralize.

4. *Am I catastrophizing?* People often exaggerate the negative significance of an event for their well-being. For example, Jane thinks that it is horrible that Ted wants to break up with her, when, in fact, although it is bad and disappointing, it is *not horrible*. She assumes that she cannot stand it, when, in fact,

it is tolerable and she is perfectly capable of coping with the disappointment and moving on with her life. To avoid this type of mistake, take a step back, take a deep breath, and ask yourself if this situation *truly* is a catastrophe (that will ruin your entire life) or, rather, a situation that is distressing and difficult, but not a catastrophe.

5. *Am I always blaming myself? Am I always blaming others?* People often incorrectly blame or judge themselves for always causing negative events that are, in fact, normal or inevitable events in life. For example, Peter usually blames himself when problems occur and assumes he is incompetent, when, in fact, no one is perfect—we all make mistakes. Others often put the entire responsibility on another's shoulders. For example, consider Anita who blames everyone else, like Jack, for not loving her and assumes that he is a bad person, when, in fact, *no one is loved by everyone.* Ask yourself such questions—do I usually think problems are my fault? Do I generally think my problems are caused by others? Both types of thinking mistakes generally lead to inaccurate problem definitions.

Do you make any of these thinking mistakes? It may be helpful to write down these questions in your notebook or journal so that you can refer to them when attempting to accurately define a problem.

## SETTING REALISTIC GOALS

In setting goals, it is important to remember to identify ones that are actually *attainable*. This means that they have to be reasonable. Although we will never discourage you from following your dreams, unless goals are reachable, you are unlikely to be able to solve most problems. Expecting yourself to complete unrealistic goals only sets you up for failure. Clinical research has repeatedly shown that a major reason why people get depressed is that they set too high goals for themselves and are never able to reach them. If a goal seems too large to try to accomplish for now, following the simplification principle, it is likely that you should break the problem down into smaller ones, while still keeping your final destination in mind. For example, setting the goal of attaining financial independence by next year is likely to be out of most people's reach. However, by stating that you wish to decrease your overall expenses in order to save an additional 5% of your salary by the end of one year appears more manageable and certainly in the right direction.

It is also important to understand the difference between problem-focused goals and emotion-focused goals. *Problem-focused goals* are objectives that involve changing the nature of a situation so that it is no longer a problem. Such goals are more appropriate for situations where the situation *can,* in fact, be changed, for example, saving more money, improving communication, or losing weight. On the other hand, *emotion-focused goals* are objectives where a situation *cannot* be changed or where one's emotional reaction, if unchanged, would create more problems in the long run. For example, fear that one may never be able to get a job that is satisfying, while understandable, is likely to cause more harm than good if unchecked. Holding onto resentment, anger, or jealousy, are other examples.

Therefore, when setting goals, you need to think about which types of goals are appropriate for the problem you are trying to deal with. Let's go back to Sam. One of the things he *can't* change is the fact that he was divorced and that some aspects of his social life have changed, such as going out as a foursome with Bill and his wife.

Because he can't be married to his ex-wife again, that part of the situation is unchangeable (although he may meet someone in the future). However, decreasing his frustration, embarrassment, and view of himself as a failure as negative emotional reactions he has about being alone are appropriate and important *emotion-focused goals* for him to consider. So is the goal of accepting that his marriage is really over. In addition, his current difficulties with his friend might be possible to change. So, having his friend more relaxed around him and less avoidant to share stories about his own wife and family can be appropriate *problem-focused goals* as well. This example illustrates the notion that most problems in life that are stressful usually involve many different goals, both emotion-focused *and* problem-focused ones.

## IDENTIFYING THE OBSTACLES TO OVERCOME

Now that you identified realistic goals, the next important question to answer is—What makes this situation a problem? In other words, what is currently preventing me from reaching such goals? This is the key question to answer in order to help us correctly define the problem. Usually problems involve obstacles to overcome or conflicts to resolve. We may not have sufficient resources or knowledge to reach a goal or there may be too many goals to choose from. As with most of life's more difficult problems, there are usually multiple factors that exist that contribute to the problem. Identifying such factors helps us to reach realistic goals. Sometimes if a problem feels very overwhelming, it is likely that we need to break it down into a set of smaller problems and tackle the various obstacles one at a time (remember the simplification principle).

For Sam, one of his obstacles was to overcome his quick trigger of anger whenever he felt frustrated. He was also experiencing conflicting goals—on one hand, he did want to have his friend's support and wanted his friendship. On the other hand, he wanted to feel that he wasn't becoming a burden and that Bill *wanted* to spend time with him. However, he also wanted to remain honest and be able to tell Bill when he was feeling upset about his divorce.

To correctly define a problem, we should answer the following questions:

- What present conditions are unacceptable (what is)?
- What changes or additions are demanded or desired (what should be)?
- What obstacle(s) exist that limit my ability to go from *A* to *B* (i.e., what makes it a problem?)

What often makes a situation a problem includes:

- *Obstacles*—something blocking your path to a goal.
- *Conflicting goals*—conflicts between yourself and others or regarding two opposing goals you have.
- *Reduced resources*—lack of necessary skills or resources that makes reaching your goal very difficult.
- *The unknown or unfamiliar*—a situation you haven't encountered before makes it difficult to know what to do.
- *Complexity*—the situation seems very complicated and overwhelming.
- *Emotional difficulties*—your emotional reaction itself is difficult to overcome.

Continuing to view yourself as a problem-solving traveler, the question to specifically ask yourself is—"What is preventing me from getting from *A* (where I am now) to *B* (where I want to go)? At this time, go back to the problem you are working on in your journal and write down what you think are any obstacles, conflicting goals, complexities, lack of resources, emotional difficulties, or unknown/unfamiliar aspects that make your situation a problem. In other words, what kind of roadblocks, long tunnels, expensive tolls, winding roads, or dangerous hills do you need to take into account when planning your trip to get to your destination? In doing so, remember to use clear language and to separate facts from assumptions.

## Remember: Correctly Defining the Problem Involves the Following Five Steps:

- Seeking the available facts
- Describing the facts in clear language
- Separating facts from assumptions
- Setting realistic goals
- Identifying the obstacles to overcome

To help you define the problem you are currently working on, we suggest that you use the format contained in the *Problem Definition Worksheet* as described below. Take out your journal or notebook once again and write down your answers for each of the four categories. Try using the worksheet now to better define your problem and set realistic goals. If working with a counselor, you may want to ask for some additional help and guidance in completing this task. Try this same task with other problems that you are experiencing, whether small or large. Write all of your answers in your journal using the same headings.

## Problem Definition Worksheet

1. *What are the facts?* Write down the facts concerning your problem. Remember to separate facts from assumptions. For example, if you experience many arguments with your spouse or significant other, state this clearly as a fact, such as "my partner and I are experiencing increased arguments about...." rather than stating an assumption, such as "my partner does not care about me."
2. *Why is this problem important to you?* If you are unable to improve this situation or the way you are feeling, what are the consequences? Why is this an important problem for you to improve? How will improving this problem improve your life (even in a small way)?
3. *What are your goals?* Be sure to make them realistic and attainable. Start with small goals that are steps to your larger goals. For example, if you want to improve your communication with your partner, a first goal might be to decrease arguments by 50% or increase the quality time alone to communicate by one hour per week.
4. *What are the major obstacles to your goal?* What is actually getting in the way of your ability to work toward your goals?

With regard to the example in number 1, possible examples of obstacles might include: you may not know how to communicate calmly or assertively without some guidance; your partner may be unavailable to you; you may lack confidence or hope.

## IF I KNOW WHAT I WANT, WHY SHOULD I DO ALL THESE STEPS?

It may seem like we are asking you to put in lots of extra work at this point, especially if you can easily state what you want, that is, your destination on your road map. Before you dismiss this task, however, answer the following question: in a game of golf, if two people have the same skills, who is more likely to eventually get a hole-in-one, the person who looks for the flag near the hole, estimates the direction of the wind, and carefully selects the correct golf club, *or* the person who swings hard, but aimlessly at the hole?

The same thing is true when trying to understand the complex and difficult problems that many of us face in the course of a lifetime. Scientific research has found that the wise old saying noted at the beginning of the chapter *is* really true—that is, a problem well-defined *is* a problem half-solved.

## REMEMBER TO HOLD OFF THINKING ABOUT SOLUTIONS OR ACTIONS TOWARD YOUR GOAL

One of the most common problems people experience when they begin to apply problem-solving principles to their everyday life is to *describe a solution rather than define a problem*. For example, consider Jane, who was under lots of stress on her job. Her boss gave her assignments that were rarely given to others. As a result, she felt that he was taking advantage of her and consequently felt overwhelmed with resentment. When Jane first tried to define the problem, she stated, "How do I let my boss know that I don't appreciate such bad treatment? " Although she deserved credit for trying to tackle this difficult and stressful problem, criticizing his way of running the office (as described above) with her boss may be one possible alternative solution, but is not a clear description of the problem. When Jane was able to stay focused on *defining* the problem, she took the time to state the facts, separate them out from assumptions, and clarify her goals and obstacles. Let's take a look at her *Problem Definition Worksheet*.

## JANE'S PROBLEM DEFINITION WORKSHEET

**The Problem:** I am very dissatisfied with work. I work hard and do a good job, but I often have to do other people's work and get many more assignments than my coworkers. I stay late and have more responsibilities than my job specifies. Sometimes I would like to have an opportunity to do extra work or help others (or not), but I would like to have compensation (either money or some other reward) for my additional work.

    **Why this is a problem for me:** I have always been willing to work hard, but people seem to take advantage of me. I end up doing work for everyone else and they don't appreciate it. Meanwhile, it's difficult for me to pursue things that I want to do for myself, like volunteer at my church, because I'm just too tired from work.

    **Realistic Goals:** I want to do my job and not constantly have my boss demand more from me; I want my coworkers not to resent me when I can't help them do their work. I want to keep my job secure, but also use my spare time to do some things that bring me joy.

    **Obstacles:** I get easily hurt when I think someone does not appreciate me. I don't know how to be assertive with my boss and set limits or ask for compensation for doing additional work. I am afraid to try because he may get angry and make me feel guilty. When I get upset at work, I am afraid that I will cry and draw negative attention from others.

    In her attempt to correctly define the problem, Jane now focused on what was currently going on, rather than what to do about it. Using the more objective and comprehensive description, there are likely to be many more alternative ways to solve this problem beyond the one where Jane tells her boss that she does not like the way he operates the office. Therefore, it is important to define the problem *before* you attempt to solve it.

## BEWARE OF SELF-PROCLAIMED EXPERTS

How many times have you discussed a problem with a friend or family member, only to be told, "*The problem is....*" or "*Here's what you have to do...*?" The fact of the matter is that many people, simply because they may have experienced something remotely similar to the problem that you are experiencing, think that they are experts in how your problem should be solved. Just think of the last time you told someone that you were shopping for a place to live, experiencing some physical symptoms, or recently had an argument with a friend. You probably got an earful of advice. It's at times like this that the self-proclaimed experts come out in full force to give you their wisdom. Real experts, such as psychologists or other professionals who have studied effective problem solving, know that no one else is an expert concerning *your* life. *You* know what your goals are, the values that you hold most important, and the resources, talents, and skills that you have. Yet, when we are under stress, it may feel good if we can avoid the hard work of problem solving and let someone else tell us what to do. Unfortunately, their opinion might represent something that is an accurate problem description for *them,* but an incorrect understanding of *your* problem. You should feel free to hear what others have to say as possible information to consider, but only *you* are the best expert on you. That is why professional therapists rarely tell people what their problem is or what they must do. Instead they take the time to understand what is important to people and then help guide them to use skills such as problem solving to help reach their own personal goals.

## HAVE YOUR FEELINGS CHANGED ABOUT WANTING TO SOLVE THIS PROBLEM?

Sometimes, once a problem has been clearly defined, individuals may no longer be as distressed or concerned about the situation as compared to when it was still vague and undefined. If so, then it may be helpful to reappraise the problem at this time. You can do this by conducting a simple cost-benefit analysis. Essentially, consider both the benefits and costs involved in solving this problem, as compared to *not* solving the problem. Consider possible *immediate* benefits and costs, possible *long-term* benefits and costs, as well as benefits and costs to *yourself* and to *significant others.*

Write these benefits and costs down on in your journal or notebook. Make two columns on a page, listing potential benefits and costs associated with *not* solving the problem in a left-hand column, and listing possible benefits and costs associated if a given goal *is obtained* in the right-hand column. Compare such consequences and use this cost-benefit analysis to reappraise the problem with regard to your well-being.

One outcome is that you might reappraise this situation as no longer being a problem that you have to solve. On the other hand, having better defined the problem might lead to a situation where you now perceive it as more threatening to your well-being. If so, ask yourself the question—"Where's the threat?" and "What's the worst thing that can happen?" Think about whether you are focusing on the *facts* or unknowingly continuing to engage in the types of thinking mistakes described earlier (for example, magnification) that are leading you to feel more threatened. Alternatively, it is possible that by better defining the problem, you have been able to identify a deeper, more complex problem that is in need of special attention. For example, Anthony, a patient we worked with, continued to define his problem as "having difficulties meeting the right person to marry." Upon continued discussions and having him complete various *Problem Definition Worksheets*, it became evident that his real problem was one of fear of intimate relationships, where he usually found fault with every woman he met and eventually sabotaged the success of these relationships in order to avoid intimacy. Therefore, all of his attempts to find the right person always failed. For Anthony, the problem was eventually more accurately defined as "How can I overcome my fears of being in a close and loving relationship with a woman?"

When you feel confident that you have learned these problem-definition skills, it is time to go on to the next chapter, that is learning how to creatively think of differing alternative solutions (Step 3 to becoming an effective problem solver).

# Step 3: Being Creative and Generating <u>A</u>lternative Solutions

## *(ad<u>A</u>pt)*

Nothing is more dangerous than an idea,
When it's the only one you have.

*—Emile Cartier*

### CONSIDER ALL THE POSSIBLE
### ROUTES ON YOUR JOURNEY

Now that you have practiced defining problems, especially with regard to the ones you are currently working to resolve, it is time to think about all the various ways you can overcome the obstacles in order to reach your problem-solving goals. If we continue to think of problem solving as a journey, reaching your goals can be thought of as getting from A to B; in other words, reaching your goals at destination B. As in any journey, even if you are clear about where you want to go, there might be several paths or roads to take to reach B. Often, there are different consequences related to taking different paths—one might be longer but cost less money, another might be more expensive but is quicker, and yet another might be more scenic, yet takes more time.

Not only are there differing consequences associated with differing alternatives, but think of having only one route to take. Think how you would feel if there were only one cereal to choose from the next time you went to the grocery store or if there were only one movie listed in the entire town where you live to go to this coming weekend. Research continues to document that when a person is only able to see a very limited number of alternatives to choose from in life, he or she is likely to experience higher levels of hopelessness and helplessness. At its extreme, such tunnel vision can lead to suicidal thoughts and behavior. As the French philosopher Cartier suggested, having only one idea can be a dangerous situation. Conversely, when we feel that have a lot of choices, we tend to feel more in control, safe, and full of hope.

Therefore, with real-life stressful problems, it is generally a good idea to think of a *variety* of ways to solve the problem, not only in order to eventually arrive at the best solution, but also to feel more hopeful. We refer to this step of problem solving as generating alternative solutions. The task at hand here is to creatively think of a comprehensive list of possible ideas. To accomplish this, we suggest that you use a variety of *brainstorming principles*. Brainstorming helps to minimize dichotomous or "black and white" thinking. It helps to decreases one's tendency to react impulsively—if you have to think of a range of ideas, you are forced to be more reflective and planful. Brainstorming also increases your flexibility and creativity, which actually improves the quality and quantity of the solutions that you generate. Research has proven this time after time.

Using brainstorming principles also helps to discourage judging ideas while thinking about novel solutions. This becomes particularly important when you have strong emotional reactions to problem situations. Emotions can often dominate or influence thinking, such that people might rigidly think only of options that maintain their negative thoughts and feelings. When emotions do seem to become overwhelming, brainstorming can help them to get back on track. Moreover, using brainstorming techniques helps to redirect a person's time and energy to focus on the task of solving a problem. You can concentrate on productive thinking, rather than on the negative emotions that surround the problem.

*Productive thinking* involves confronting problems directly by creatively developing a list of possible ways to resolve your problems. This is in contrast to *nonproductive* thinking, which refers to thoughts *unrelated* to solving a problem, but focuses rather on emotional distress.

Consider the following differences in the reactions between Rita and Naomi, who both missed the last train home from work. Both had dinner engagements scheduled for later in the evening. Rita focuses her attention on her negative thoughts of irresponsibility, carelessness, and unreliability, as well as negative emotions of sadness and anger at herself. She also concentrates on her disappointment that the train is gone, which means that she would arrive home late causing her to miss her dinner date. She continues to lament these negative thoughts, which eventually spiral into more negative thoughts and emotions. Four hours later, Rita is still sitting at the station counting her woes. This is the result of nonproductive thinking.

On the other hand, Naomi chooses to stop and think rationally about her problem ("I have missed the train"), as well as her goal ("How can I get home as quickly as possible without ruining my evening, given that I have missed the last train?"). Following this path of productive thinking, Naomi attempts to generate a variety of alternative ways to reach her goal. Her partial list includes calling to delay her dinner date, taking a bus, taking a taxi, asking someone for a ride home, calling home and having someone pick her up, and taking a train at a different station and going straight to the restaurant to meet her dinner date rather going home first. Four hours later, we find Naomi enjoying the evening with a pleasant companion who picked her up from a different train station.

There are three brainstorming principles to use to increase your chances of ultimately identifying effective solutions:

- Quantity leads to quality
- Defer judgment
- Variety—think of strategies and tactics

## QUANTITY PRINCIPLE

This principle suggests that it is important to generate as many ideas or solution options as possible. The concept of generating numerous responses to problems, and elaborating upon these responses, is supported by research findings showing that people will improve the selection of high-quality ideas by increasing the number of alternative solutions. In addition, in keeping with the externalization rule of problem-solving multi-tasking, drafting a written list of ideas, rather than composing a list of ideas in one's head, can help people to improve both the quantity and quality of thinking. Recording ideas on paper keeps the problem solver focused on the task at hand and reduces repetition of ideas or getting stuck on the same idea. Furthermore, the written results of the brainstorming exercise can be maintained for future reference and can serve as a concrete reinforcement of one's problem-solving attempts.

Providing brief catch phrases can aid us all during attempts to use these skills. For example, we have often asked our patients the following question—"Which store is more likely to have your size and selection, a large store or a smaller store?" Obviously, we all would prefer to go to the larger store to increase our selection choices. Parenthetically, we have come across skeptical patients, who because they may be resistant to learning new techniques, have challenged this analogy. Consider, Don, a 46-year-old man, who, upon hearing the "store" analogy, retorted—"Well, that's not really true because when I went to buy my son's baseball pants, I checked out a few stores and the department store was more expensive than the little shop near our house! I saved twelve bucks!" In response, we pointed out to him, "That's great! Yet, had you never checked out *several* stores, you would have never known what a great deal you got!"

## DEFERMENT PRINCIPLE

To further facilitate brainstorming, you should *defer judgment*. This principle suggests that it is important to record *every* idea that comes to mind as a means to increase the quantity of solutions. Prematurely rejecting ideas can limit productive and creative thinking that often leads to effective solutions. Therefore, it's really important to refrain from evaluating solutions at this point in the problem-solving process. There is only one criterion to use at this time—that the idea is *relevant* to the problem at hand. Otherwise, remember that there is no right or wrong alternative at this juncture—if you catch yourself (even silently) judging any ideas you have, stop and remind yourself that this will cut down on creativity.

People are often reluctant to allow themselves to express ideas that they believe are silly, unrealistic, stupid, or could reflect badly upon them. Actually, deferring judgment increases one's effectiveness. For example, even if an idea seems silly or initially impossible, it may spark another related idea that is not silly or impossible. Some of the practice exercises that we use when working with people to improve these skills involve having people deliberately offering alternatives that might be regarded as outlandish or impractical if evaluated critically.

Some people may have difficulty adhering to the deferment-of-judgment principle. For example, several individuals we have worked with develop the "yeah, but ..." syndrome in response to their own alternatives or alternatives offered by another. We commonly hear the following—"Yeah, *but* that won't work because....," "Yeah, *but* I would never do that because....," "That sounds okay, *but* what if....," "I thought of that, *but* I didn't write it down because...." If you feel this "but" urge as well, consider the following analogy.

Think of the list you are putting together as a restaurant menu you need to prepare. On most dinner menus, there are a variety of options to please the tastes of children, adults, senior citizens, people who are very hungry, people who only want a snack, people who want late-night breakfast menus, desserts, or steak dinners. There may be some items on the menu that certain people might not enjoy, or others that they might not have thought of eating at a particular time of the day. But, by the very fact that your restaurant offers a *variety* of choices, you will be more likely to satisfy your patrons. Likewise, deferring judgment about the menu of alternative solutions you create to solve your problems will increase the likelihood that you will have a variety of choices or satisfactory ideas that will meet your goals. You may not like all of the alternatives; however, there is no harm in listing them on the menu. When you engage in decision making at a later point, you can select which solutions are best suited for you.

## VARIETY PRINCIPLE — 
## THINK OF STRATEGIES *AND* TACTICS

According to the *variety* principle, the greater the range or variety of solution alternatives generated, the more good quality ideas will be made available. When generating specific solution alternatives, some individuals develop an inclination to produce ideas that reflect only one strategy or general approach to the problem. This narrow set of ideas may occur even when you apply the quantity and deferment-of-judgment principles. To change such a perspective, peruse your list of solution alternatives after using the quantity and deferment-of-judgment principles and identify all the *different* strategies that you have. In essence, you are trying to identify differing classifications—that is, group your solution alternatives according to some common theme.

If any of the strategies have very few specific solutions, think of more specific solution alternatives for that particular strategy. Then try to think of new strategies that are not yet represented by any of the available solutions and generate additional specific solution ideas for those strategies.

Learning to differentiate between strategies and tactics can really enhance your brainstorming options. *Strategies* are general courses of action people can take to try and improve a problematic situation. For example, one woman we worked with, Sophie, described herself as "angry, sad, and hurt" following several incidents in which her daughter and son-in-law had left her out of holiday plans and special events that involved her grandchildren. She brainstormed multiple ideas in which she might communicate with her grown daughter and son-in-law regarding ways she hoped their relationship might be improved. Her goal was to communicate how important the relationship was to her and what she believed needed to take place for it to change. She listed a few general *strategies* first. These included the following, among others:

- Ignoring their acts of insensitivity
- Expressing her anger and feelings of hurt
- Inviting them to stay with her for a few days to talk

- Asking them to be kinder to her and include her in family celebrations
- Threatening to remove them from her will unless they changed
- Telling them that it is important to her to see her grandchildren
- Communicating clearly and specifically how she hopes to be treated in the future

*Tactics* are specific steps involved in putting a strategy into action. When thinking about different tactics, we encourage people to generate as many options as possible, while continuing to defer judgment. Sophie also included tactics in her list of alternatives. For example, with regard to communicating clearly and specifically how she hoped to be treated in the future, she generated the following *tactics:*

- Speak to her daughter and son-in-law in person the next time she saw them
- Make specific arrangements to discuss the matter
- Send an e-mail
- Write a letter
- Have another family member communicate her feelings
- Have someone neutral mediate the discussion
- Call them on the telephone

By providing two different ways to think of alternatives, the strategy-tactics principle often provides new viewpoints from which to originate alternative solutions. Overall problem-solving efforts are likely to be less effective or productive if limited by the use of only one strategy. Therefore, it is important to think about a wide variety of both strategies and tactics, rather than focusing on one or two narrow tactics or limiting oneself only to general approaches.

For example, Sophie was having difficulty thinking of more solutions when she realized that all of her strategies were centered on the theme of ways to get her daughter and son-in-law to change. When she realized this, she decided to try to think of other available general strategies. She realized that getting herself and her husband to change and accept their daughter's behavior as out of their control represented a whole series of other tactics that she had not previously recognized. There were many new tactics she was able to list under the category of "ways that I can change to improve the relationship." These included the following:

- Arranging her own family celebrations and events
- Communicating directly with her grandchildren
- Changing her view of their behavior to be less negative

- Asking her husband's help in setting special visits
- Reducing her expectations

## KEEPING THE CREATIVE JUICES FLOWING

As we illustrated in the previous example, Sophie found that examining her ongoing list of strategies and tactics and the realization that she was limiting her general strategies served to be an important way to stimulate her creativity and think of additional strategies. Another way to stimulate creativity when feeling stuck is to imagine how someone else may try to solve the problem. It is helpful here to think of someone whom you admire for their wisdom, strength, courage, or creativity. For example, one of Sophie's favorite television shows was "Oprah." Therefore, one way that she might be able to think of different types of strategies would be to imagine that Oprah was facing the same problem and ask herself, "What would Oprah do?" Other people might use a favorite character from a movie or a novel and imagine that they are seeing the problem through their eyes. Other people may imagine that they are having a conversation with a spiritual leader or role model, such as their favorite rabbi, the Dali Lama, or Jesus, and think what they might suggest is in the person's best interest to do. Still others might think about friends or family members and what they would do to solve the problem.

Another way is to use the visualization principle—think of the problem in your imagination, then visualize yourself attempting to cope with it and achieving your problem-solving goal. Think about differing ways to achieve such goals.

Other ways to foster your creativity are to *combine* differing ideas to produce new solution alternatives or to *modify* an alternative to either improve upon it or produce a new one.

The important point is that by using your creative juices and imagination in these ways, you gain additional perspectives and help your mind to get out of its stalled position and be able to create your own options and choices.

## PRACTICE GENERATING ALTERNATIVES

Learning any new skill requires that you first practice with easier tasks. For example, you probably did not go on a major highway the first day you learned to drive. You probably did not enter a tennis tournament the second time you took a tennis lesson. You get the idea. If generating multiple ideas proves a bit difficult for you with regard to the real-life problems you are currently experiencing, one way to improve your basic creativity skills is to practice with "fun" examples or problems that only may be hypothetical ones for you.

For instance, we often use the following example when working with groups—to generate as many ideas about what one can do with a single brick. Believe it or not, within minutes, such a list can top over 100 ideas. For fun, go ahead and try this practice example. Write down in your journal as many ideas as you possibly can within five minutes different things you can do with a single brick. If you experience some creative blocks, remember the brainstorming principles—quantity leads to quality, defer judgment, and think of various general classes of ideas (that is, strategies), as well as specific examples of these classes (that is, tactics). Think also of a role model and what he or she might do with a brick; what would Martha Stewart do with a brick? Arnold Schwarzenegger? A criminal? An artist? A gardener? Do you find these tips helpful for you to think of more ideas?

A second "fun" idea might be to think of as many things you can do with a wire hanger. A more real-life problem, perhaps one you yourself are experiencing, might be to think of as many ideas as you can to meet new people now that you moved to another neighborhood and feel isolated. Try these exercises simply to practice these skills.

Now, go back and identify a stressful situation that you previously worked on in order to come up with a well-defined problem with a set of realistic goals. In your journal or notebook, begin generating a list of possible solution alternatives to that problem. Remember to use the brainstorming principles. If you experience a block, put down your pen, go away from this task, and come back again after a few hours and try again. At times, your brain may be working on this task without you even knowing it.

## CREATIVE PEOPLE ARE NOT AFRAID OF FAILING

One of the biggest roadblocks to creativity is fear. This includes fear of not being smart enough to think of different ideas, fear of coming up with stupid or bad ideas, fear of considering alternatives that might make you feel like you are giving in to others or letting them off the hook, fear that your solution will not be perfect, and so forth. We could go on, but you probably get the idea. One thing that creative people have in common is that they are not afraid to think outside the box, do things that others don't expect or approve of, or consider alternative actions and viewpoints that are new. By continuing to think of a variety of alternatives in spite of your worries (we know that you will have them), you increase your creativity in leaps and bounds. We are reminded of an ancient saying by Confucius—"Our greatest glory is not in never falling, but in rising every time we fall." If you do experience significant emotional obstacles to being creative, go back to Chapter 5 to practice the skills involved in learning how to use your emotions more adaptively.

# CHAPTER 7

# Step 4: _P_redicting the Consequences and Developing a Solution Plan

## (ada_P_t)

There are in nature neither rewards not punishments,
There are consequences.

—*Robert Ingersoll*

If you have successfully brainstormed many possible solutions to the problem you defined earlier, you are probably wondering—With so many ideas and possibilities, how do I decide what to actually do about the problem? In other words, which of these solutions will work best for me? This chapter focuses on teaching you how to evaluate the potential effectiveness of each solution alternative that you generated by focusing on the consequences. This information is important because it gives you an idea about what to expect and can help you to determine whether you need to continue to work on the problem or if the problem is likely to be solved.

When discussing with our patients the actions they have taken in response to a problem, we have often been asked—*Was that a good thing for me to do?* The answer, of course, depends upon what their goals were and if the responses chosen were effective steps toward the outcome they wanted. When you learn how to evaluate the likely success of a given course of action, you also learn to answer this question yourself. Doing so can give you confidence to move forward.

### YOU BE THE JUDGE

Remember back to the last chapter when you were creatively thinking of many different alternatives for your problem? We strongly suggested that you *defer any judgment* as a way to help your ideas flow more freely. Now, judgment will be the central activity. You will begin to evaluate the likely success of the various options and then decide which ones to carry out. This will include thinking about all the positive and negative consequences of each alternative idea. People, especially when they're distressed, often wish to only consider how effective a solution will be in terms of taking away the problem as soon as possible. By taking a few moments to be a little bit more objective and systematic as you evaluate each idea, you stand a better chance of minimizing negative consequences and maximizing positive consequences. However, whether a consequence is positive or negative depends heavily on the situation and can differ greatly depending on who is having the problem. Once again, this is the very reason why it's important to learn effective problem-solving skills, rather than to simply be told what to do. We are all different, and the effects of the same solution plan may be different depending on who we are. As the quote by 19th-century American lawyer, Robert Ingersoll, suggested at the beginning of this chapter—consequences are neither inherently positive or negative, but exist nonetheless. It's up to us to be able to evaluate what's right for us.

## THE FALLOUT OF BAD DECISIONS

Almost anything you choose to do, or any way you choose to think about things, *is* a solution. Often, we think of solutions as *any* action taken to solve a problem. What sometimes we forget is that there are many ineffective solutions we use every day that may solve a *part* of the problem, but simultaneously also create additional problems, distress, and various negative consequences. For example, drinking, gambling, avoidance, aggressive statements and behavior, or thinking in ways to try and convince oneself of something that is not accurate are all ways that people use to try to solve problems every day. These solutions often provide some short-term relief or distraction but have many lasting negative consequences. Such actions often create further problems and the individual will eventually be left feeling additionally frustrated, hopeless, and ineffective. Everyone likes a little short-term relief from distress, but it's important to try to predict both the costs and benefits of a course of action you decide to take, as well as its impact on your overall well-being and that of others.

Effective solutions, on the other hand, not only help you get closer to your goals, but reduce the negative side effects or fallout of your decisions for the future. Sometimes effective decisions may be a bit more difficult to implement in the short term but can ultimately have so many positive short-term and long-term consequences that they are worth the extra work.

For example, a woman we worked with, Bernice, had a history of relationships in which she sacrificed herself for the needs and desires of others. In her family, although she was the only person who had a full-time job, she frequently accommodated her plans to the whim of her aging parents who lived nearby. When she wanted to move away from them to take a better-paying job, she received little support. Her parents complained—"Who would take us to doctors' appointments or family get-togethers?" Bernice had a long pattern of blaming herself and believing that she had to always please others, even though her partner, Jana, tried hard to convince her to become more independent. She was also very grateful that her parents were always supportive of her relationship with Jana. Therefore, in trying to cope with this problem, one of Bernice's initial solution alternatives was *"to convince my partner, Jana, that the move and the new job isn't so important—I'd rather stay put so I don't have to deal with guilt from my family, after all, they are supportive of us!"* However, Jana often felt frustrated watching others take advantage of Bernice's generous nature and was angry that her family was not supportive of the move, especially since it meant a significant boost for her career. Unfortunately, Bernice often fought with Jana and secretly wished she could just do what her parents wanted so she could just avoid the whole matter. However, the more that Bernice considered this alternative, the more she realized that there were many long-term consequences to choosing this option. For one, she was missing out on an important and well-paying job. In addition, there were consequences for her relationship with Jana. Finally, her family members were unlikely to change and no matter how much she thought "Well, there's always next time," she did realize that she could expect to continually face the same problem over and over again. As Bernice became more creative in generating alternatives, she discovered that there were other ways she could objectively be a resource to her parents, but without having to sacrifice her career and her own happiness.

## MAKING EFFECTIVE DECISIONS

Making decisions about what to do to solve your difficult problems can be hard. As Irish novelist, George Moore, once said—"The difficulty in life is the choice." However, even though making decisions can be tough, it can lead to more control over our lives and enhanced well-being.

Research has shown that there are four important steps to making effective decisions:

- Screening out obviously ineffective solutions
- Predicting possible consequences

- Evaluating solution outcomes
- Identifying effective solutions and developing a solution plan

## Rough Screening of Solution Alternatives

Making a decision about which ideas are potentially the best can be made easier if you first conduct a "rough screening" of the list of possible alternatives in order to eliminate any that are clearly inferior. Remember that the only criteria that should have been used while generating alternatives is that they are *relevant* to the problem at hand. Therefore, it is possible that if you tried to use the brainstorming principles, several ineffective ideas were likely to have been generated. Therefore, rather than spending time going through to rate each alternative, it is a good idea to conduct such an initial screening. At this point, eliminate any alternatives that are clearly ineffective, that is, ones that (a) are likely to create serious negative consequences, or (b) are very difficult to implement.

## Predicting Consequences

When predicting the consequences of a given alternative, first think of the following two questions:

- Will this solution help me reach my goals?
- Will I be able to carry it out?

Next, predict the consequences of each alternative according to various *personal* and *social* consequences as noted below. Be sure to think of both *short-term* and *long-term* consequences in each category.

*Personal consequences,* that is, the effects on you, the problem solver, that should be considered include the following:

1. Effects on emotional well-being (pleasure versus pain)
2. Time and effort expended
3. Effects on physical well-being
4. Effects on psychological well-being (for example, depression, anxiety, self-esteem)
5. Effects on economic well-being (for example, job security)
6. Self-enhancement (for example, achievements, knowledge)
7. Effects on other personal goals, values, and commitments

*Social consequences,* that is, the effects on others, include:

1. Effects on the personal and/or social well-being of significant others
2. Effects on the rights of others

3. Effects on significant interpersonal relationships
4. Effects on personal and/or social performance evaluations (e.g., reputation, status, prestige)

Looking over these checklists, you probably realize that solutions for real-life problems are likely to have many different consequences. Remembering the externalization rule of problem-solving multi-tasking, therefore, it is important to write down the major significant expected consequences (for example, Bernice might write—"I am likely to feel very guilty; my parents will be very hurt; in the long run I could mess up my relationship with Jana; I could lose this job opportunity"). This will help you to better identify all of the possible consequences, both positive and negative, of a given action.

## Evaluating Solution Outcomes

This task suggests that you rate each alternative according to the various consequences you previously identified. To help you accomplish this task more systematically, it would be important to write your ratings down. Therefore, get out your journal or notebook now. At the top of the page, write down your problem-solving goal. Next, write an abbreviated form of each alternative you previously generated. If you have been working on a particular problem in each of the previous chapters thus far, go back and get this information from previous exercises (that is, defining a problem, generating alternatives). However, if you wish to work on a different problem, you need to go back and engage in Steps 2 and 3.

Now, on the right hand side of the page, make four columns, one to represent your answers to each of the following four questions (see sample worksheet):

1. Will this solution solve the problem?
2. Can I *really* carry it out?
3. What are the overall effects on myself, both short-term and long-term?
4. What are the overall effects on others, both short-term and long-term?

After you conduct a rough screening of the entire list of alternatives as suggested previously, for each alternative, go through all of these four questions and rate each alternative using the following rating scale:

+ = *generally positive*   – = *generally negative*   0= *neutral*

When rating an alternative, seriously consider each of the four questions. Think about the consequences. If the answer, for example, for a given alternative to the first question (will it solve my problem?) is yes, then place a plus sign (+) in that column. If your answer is probably not, than place a minus sign (−) in that column, and so forth. Do this with every alternative for each of the four questions.

At times it may not be easy to predict and evaluate specific consequences of solutions before they are experienced, especially subjective consequences such as feelings and emotions. If this occurs, try to visualize what would happen if you carried out a particular solution option. Focus on your thoughts and feelings. Try to actually "experience" the consequences. Jot them down in your notebook. Now look them over and reconsider your ratings.

## Identifying Effective Solutions and Developing a Solution Plan

After you rated each alternative, ask yourself the following three questions:

1. Is the problem solvable? (i.e., "Is there a satisfactory solution?")
2. Do I need more information before I can select a solution to carry out?
3. What solution or solution combination should I choose to implement?

*Is the Problem Solvable?* Answering this question requires that you begin to add up the ratings that you have for each alternative (that is, how many plusses, how many minuses, and how many zero's). If you are able to identify effective solutions, then the answer is yes. In other words, effective alternatives are those with the least number of negative consequences (fewer minuses) and the most number of positive consequences (more plusses). However, when making this evaluation, keep in mind that *no* solution is perfect. If your alternative solutions with the highest ratings still have some negative consequences that are likely to occur, you may want to look over the other alternatives you listed and see if you have any alternatives that did not have the same negative effects. Some people have found that through this process, they are able to think about how to slightly change or adjust the highest rated alternative to further reduce the negative consequences associated with it. However, it is important to remember that it may not be possible to reduce *all* negative consequences. Effective problem solvers reduce negative consequences as much as possible but know that there are always likely to be some possible side effects of any solution.

*Do I need more information before I can select a solution or solution combination for implementation?* If it turns out that most of your alternatives appear to be rated as rather negative (that is, associated with a lot of minuses), then it is possible that you need to step back and reconsider whether you correctly defined the problem and/or generated sufficient numbers of alternatives. If so, then go back and engage in either or both steps once again. However, another possibility exists when there are very few potentially effective solution ideas—you may now realize, after thinking a lot about various solutions and their effects, that in fact this problem is *not* solvable. If so, then you may need to reconsider your goals and change them to ones that are more *emotion-focused* (for example, changing your reaction to the problem; accepting that the situation cannot be changed the way you would like) rather than attempting to solve an unsolvable problem.

*What solution or solution combination should I choose to implement?* At this point, you should choose alternatives that have the best ratings in order to develop a *solution plan*. In keeping with our definition of an *effective solution,* your solution plan should be consistent with the general goal of resolving the problem satisfactorily, while maximizing positive consequences and minimizing negative effects.

A solution plan may be *simple* or *complex*. For a simple plan, based on your ratings, you can choose a single solution or course of action. When there is one solution that you predict will lead to a highly satisfactory outcome, a simple plan may be enough. However, sometimes more difficult problems require a more complex solution plan. There are two types of complex plans—a *solution combination* and a *contingency plan*. For a solution combination, you can choose a *combination* of solution alternatives to be carried out at the same time. Do this when it seems that such a combination is likely to be more effective than any solution alone or when there are several obstacles that need to be overcome. As many problems in life are complex and involve multiple obstacles to overcome prior to effective problem resolution, identifying several specific solution tactics to include in a larger solution plan is advisable. *Contingency plans* involve choosing a combination of solutions to be implemented contingently—that is, implement solution A first; if that does not work, implement solution B; if that does not work, carry out solution C, and so forth.

Another type of contingency plan occurs when you first implement a particular course of action, A, and, then, depending on the outcome of A, you carry out either B or C. Use such a contingency plan when you are rather uncertain about the exact effects of any one solution or solution combination. In that case, it is advisable to have a contingency plan to save time in case the initial solution choice is unsuccessful.

Once the solution plan has been prepared, the final step before carrying it out is to fill in the details as to exactly how, when, and where it will be implemented.

## PRACTICE EXAMPLE

As a possible example to practice these decision-making skills, try to solve the following problem. In doing so, you will be able to build up your skills when you are trying to solve your own problems.

## Problem

You and your family are driving to a movie, but running late. You see that you are low on gas. You might be able to make it to the theater without stopping, and yet, looking at the time, if you do stop, you will probably be late. On the other hand, you may not have enough gas to get to the theater. What do you do?

## Problem-Solving Goal

To have a nice evening with your family watching a movie

## Possible Alternatives (as Listed in Sample Decision-Making Worksheet)

- Do not stop, and keep driving to the movie
- Stop for gas
- Forget about the movie for tonight
- Stop and call AAA
- Go to a restaurant closer to where you are now
- Go to a shopping mall instead
- Call a friend to bring gas to you
- Park the car and call for a taxi
- and so forth (for practice in generating alternatives, you may wish to use the brainstorming principles to think of more ideas)

## SAMPLE DECISION-MAKING WORKSHEET

| ALTERNATIVES | Q1 | Q2 | Q3 | Q4 |
|---|---|---|---|---|
| Do not stop, and keep driving to the movie | | | | |
| Stop for gas | | | | |
| Forget about the movie for tonight | | | | |
| Stop and call AAA | | | | |
| Go to a restaurant closer to where you are now | | | | |
| Go to a shopping mall instead | | | | |
| Call a friend to bring gas to you | | | | |
| Park the car and call for a taxi | | | | |

## Predicting Consequences

As an example, let's consider the first idea—*Do not stop, and keep driving to the movie.*

For now, try practicing how to identify, predict, and evaluate the hypothetical effects that might occur if *you* were experiencing this problem. Write down the various consequences in your journal or notebook and then evaluate each one. As an example, note what one person we worked with, Fred, wrote down in terms of possible consequences:

- *Effects on me*—feel very anxious while driving; exhausted from walking if we run out of gas; feel bad for getting family stuck; feel angry with myself for not stopping earlier (an important value I have for myself is being better prepared); we may not get to the movie if car runs out of gas; we may have to walk for gas; I don't know where the nearest station is; I might feel relieved if we make it to the movie in time; gas station may not be open after movie.

- *Effects on others*—family would be scared and upset if we don't make it; family would be happy if we make it to movie in time; I set a bad example for my kids being unprepared.

This example has no perfect answer, of course, but it is designed to give you practice in predicting consequences and rating alternatives and seeing that most alternatives lead to *some* positive and *some* negative consequences. Good decisions are those that involve solutions with more positive consequences than negative. Sometimes, taking the time to identify all the different types of effects of any given alternative can trigger ideas that allow us to go back and actually list a few additional options.

For additional practice, try working on another one of your own problems that you would like to resolve. Go through problem-solving Steps 1, 2, and 3, that is, try to adopt a positive attitude toward solving it, define it correctly and set realistic goals, and generate a variety of solution options. Now predict the consequences for each and rate the alternatives. Based on these ratings, identify the most effective ones and develop an overall solution plan.

## DO I NEED TO GO THROUGH THIS ENTIRE PROCEDURE EACH TIME I AM TRYING TO MAKE A DECISION?

It depends! Going through each specific step in this decision-making task at this point is similar to driving in a deserted parking lot on a Sunday morning while you are learning how to drive. In other words, the more you practice each step, the more likely each will become more automatic for you. As such, the more you practice predicting and rating the value of the various consequences, the more likely you are to do so in the future without having to construct such a table each time you wish to solve a personal problem. However, many of our former patients have told us that when it came to very difficult or complex problems, going through each step was very helpful in ultimately developing an effective solution plan.

Now that you have developed a solution plan, go on to Step five in the next chapter—"Trying out the solution in real-life."

# CHAPTER 8

# Step 5: <u>T</u>rying Out Your Solution Plan and Determining If It Works

## *(adap<u>T</u>)*

The sweetest part is action
After making a decision.

*—Indigo Girls*

There are costs and risks to a program of action,
but they are far less than the long range risks and costs of comfortable inaction.

*—John F. Kennedy*

As the song by the Indigo Girls suggests, after making a decision, it will probably feel good to carry out your solution plan. However, doing so is *not* the end of the story. Too often, once we make a decision and implement our action plan, we stop being systematic and planful. In order to be an effective problem solver, there is yet one more part to this last step—to monitor and evaluate the actual success of the solution plan *after it is carried out.* This is important in order to (a) determine whether you need to continue to work on the problem or if the problem is actually successfully resolved, and (b) understand what areas, if any, of your problem-solving skills require some additional fine tuning.

### YOUR PROBLEM-SOLVING OUTCOME WILL NOT ALWAYS BE PERFECT

We thought that we should reemphasize this healthy thinking rule because some people continue to hold unrealistically high expectations for themselves. We have frequently heard people say, *"but I really tried hard and it still didn't turn out the way I wanted it to."* Remember when we first talked about a good problem-solving attitude? Part of being an effective problem solver is to keep your expectations *realistic*. In addition, it is important to focus on the positive consequences, rather than only on the negative effects.

## STEPS TO TRYING OUT YOUR SOLUTION

This final step in the problem-solving process suggests that you engage in the following activities:

- Motivate yourself to carry out your solution
- Implement your action plan
- Observe and monitor your results
- Reward yourself for your problem-solving efforts
- Trouble-shoot areas of difficulty
- Know when to get professional help

## MOTIVATE YOURSELF TO CARRY OUT YOUR SOLUTION PLAN

Although you probably have already spent significant energy engaging in the previous four steps of effective problem solving (that is, adopting a positive attitude, defining your problem accurately and realistically, brainstorming strategies and tactics concerning ways to improve the problem, predicting and weighing the various costs and benefits of each solution's likely effects, and selecting a course of action), you still have to carry out your solution. Think of your solution plan now as your *action plan,* that is, your solution needs to be put into action. However, occasionally we might get fearful or concerned about taking action, either because of what it means about changes in ourselves (for example, changing our own attitudes) or changing the nature of the problem situation itself (for example, trying to change others' behavior or certain situations). At such times it may be important to try to motivate yourself to actually carry out your action plan. Remember the worksheet that you completed during Step 2 of problem solving after you defined a problem? At that time, you were asked to conduct a simple cost-benefit analysis of consequences that might occur if your feelings about wanting to solve the problem had changed. At this time, you should complete a similar worksheet to help remind yourself of the importance of changing even seemingly small problems and to increase your motivation to carry your problem-solving efforts through this final stage.

## Motivational Worksheet

Take out your journal or notebook once again. Make two columns on a page, listing potential benefits and costs associated with *not* solving the problem in the left-hand column, and listing possible benefits and costs associated if a given goal *is obtained* in the right-hand column. Compare such consequences and use this cost-benefit analysis to reappraise the problem with regard to your well-being. Remember to consider possible *immediate* benefits and costs, and possible *long-term* benefits and costs, as well as benefits and costs to *yourself* and to *significant others*. After you have made the list, you may want to post this motivational worksheet in your home or office to continually remind yourself of why you chose to focus on this problem and worked so hard to discover a solution in the first place. Note the late President Kennedy's words at the beginning of this chapter that suggest that although there are risks associated with any plan of action, there are more serious consequences associated with *inaction*.

## Additional Obstacles to Trying Out Your Solution

Even if you are very eager to carry out your action plan, at times you may experience unexpected obstacles. For example, the problem may have gotten worse over time or you experienced a decrease in your resources. As such, although you might feel motivated to carry out your plan, you remain anxious or worried. You may also realize that your plan requires certain knowledge or abilities that you really do not possess at this time. If carrying out your plan is not possible or feasible at this juncture for such reasons, you can:

- Return to previous steps in the problem-solving process in order to identify an alternative solution that may be implemented more effectively, or
- Use the five problem-solving steps to help overcome these newly discovered obstacles.

If emotional barriers continue to exist, go to the exercises and activities described in Chapter 5 and included in the appendices (stress management strategies) to help you manage your emotions more effectively.

## CARRY OUT YOUR SOLUTION

Now is the time to launch your solution plan. When you used your decision-making skills to select which alternative seemed to be the best match for your current problem, you also developed an action plan regarding how you would carry it out (for example, you may have decided to develop a simple or complex plan, a solution combination, or a contingency plan). This is particularly important, because even with the most creative and useful ideas, it is important to have a step-by-step plan of how you will put your ideas into action. It is important to have the steps in your plan written down so you can check off each part of the plan and observe the results as you carry out your solution.

For example, remember one of our patients, Jane, from Chapter 6, who was experiencing a problem with her boss at work. Jane's problem-solving goals were to be recognized and compensated for the work she was expected to do that was beyond the requirements of her job as a secretary for a public television news station. For example, in addition to the secretarial duties that defined her job, she was often planning and managing special events, preparing promotional articles about the station for their public education campaign, and helping the station associate producer with managing the volunteer staff. After generating and rating many alternatives to help reach her goals, Jane selected the alternative of arranging a special meeting with her boss to request a raise.

Her plan included:

- Setting up the meeting during the time that budgets were being decided.
- Making this appointment with her boss at the end of the day on a Monday (Mondays, in general, were less hectic and there was less stress present in the station).
- Making a list of the work that she completed that was in excess of her position.
- Estimating the financial benefits to the station for her additional work (for example, successfully organizing the volunteers, the amount of donations received after a successful event, etc.).

In addition, to help her carry out this plan optimally, Jane asked her cousin, Kerry, who worked for a human resources department for a large local company, to role-play the meeting with her and give her tips and feedback on the words and behavior that might help get her points across effectively. Jane then made a list of everything she needed to do to optimally carry out her plan, so she would able to monitor the effects of each step along the way.

## Aids to Help Carry Out Your Solution Plan Optimally

In order to increase the likelihood that you are able to carry out your action plan in its most optimal fashion, here are some additional tips:

- Rehearse the plan in your imagination before you carry it out.
- Like Jane, role-play the action plan with someone you trust.
- Think the plan out loud (for example, "First I need to state my goals and think about the positive consequences that will occur when I solve this problem. Now I need to take a deep breath and go ahead and carry out the solution. When I begin talking to my boss, I realize that I might get anxious, so I need to practice what I might say to him right before I see him. Then I will remind myself to speak calmly and deliberately so I don't get more nervous....").
- Write down the steps in detail, similar to an instruction or user's manual.

## MONITOR THE OUTCOME

If you are trying to lose weight, it makes sense to weigh yourself on a weekly basis. If you are trying to save additional money, it makes sense to balance your checkbook and keep sales receipts. If you are trying to lower your high blood pressure, it makes sense to go for routine physicals. The same is true for problem solving. As such, it is important to monitor both your actual performance in carrying out the solution, as well as the outcome. There are several possible ways to record such information—the type of measure that is most appropriate for a particular problem depends on the type of behavior or action plan that you are evaluating. Examples include the following.

### Response Frequency

You simply count the number of responses. Examples include the number of cigarettes smoked, the number of times a child gets out of his or her seat or talks out of turn in class, the number of times a teenage daughter violates curfew, or the number of requests you make for a date.

### Response Duration

You can also record the amount of time it takes to perform a response. For example, the time it takes to complete a report, time spent studying, time spent exercising each day, time spent commuting to work, and time spent sleeping.

### Response Latency

You can also record the time between the occurrence of a particular event and the onset of a particular response. For example, the number of minutes late to class, the amount of time beyond curfew, the amount of time late for dinner, or the amount of time a child takes to get a job done following a request.

### Response Intensity

You might be able to rate the degree of intensity of something, such as the degree of anxiety, the intensity or severity of a headache, the degree of depression, the intensity of sexual arousal, or the degree of pleasure or satisfaction associated with a particular activity. This can often be accomplished using a simple rating scale, for example, such as 1 to 5, where 1 = little to no anxiety, and 5 = severe anxiety.

### Response Product

This involves the *by-products* or *effects* of a behavior. Examples include the number of dates accepted, the number of boxes packed per hour, the number of sales made, the number of chapters studied, the number of arrests made, and the number of problems solved.

Take out your notebook or journal and write down some ideas for how you will monitor and evaluate the outcome of your solution (remember to use brainstorming principles to develop creative ways of doing so that suit your needs).

## GIVE YOURSELF A PERFORMANCE EVALUATION

If you have carefully observed each step of your plan and monitored the results along the way, you will be able to actually rate your performance after putting your plan into action. As an example, Jane observed that she experienced significant anxiety and fear thinking that asking for financial recognition would seem too "pushy" (she was always hesitant to assert herself). However, she discovered that listing out the actual financial benefits of her work was helpful to her to better realize and accept her own value to the station. As such, Jane actually found it a bit easier (although she was still anxious) to ask for increased compensation. In addition, she was able to see that until she worked with her cousin to practice what she would say, she was not feeling very confident. However, the role-play practice and advice from her cousin helped her to develop a script with which she felt more comfortable.

Take out your journal and using the questions contained in the *Performance Evaluation Worksheet* below to guide your self-evaluation, write down your actual ratings of both your own performance and the results you achieved in carrying out your plan.

## Performance Evaluation Worksheet

Using a scale from 1 to 5, where *1* = not at all, *3* = somewhat, and *5* = very much, answer the following questions:

1.  How satisfactory are the results of your solution plan?
2.  How well did your solution plan meet your goals?
3.  How satisfied were you with the effects on you?
4.  How well did these effects match your original predictions about personal consequences?
5.  How satisfied were you with the impact on others?
6.  How well did these results match your original predictions about the consequences concerning others?
7.  Overall, how satisfied are you with the results?

Based on the answers to these questions, is the match between what you expected and what actually happened a good one? In other words:

- Was the problem solved?
- Was the effect on you more positive than negative?
- Was the effect on others more positive than negative?

If the answers to these questions are essentially yes, than go to the very next step, the one that suggests you reward yourself!

## REWARD YOURSELF FOR YOUR PROBLEM-SOLVING EFFORTS

Now is the time to reward yourself for your problem-solving efforts. Please note that we did *not* indicate that you should confine your self-reward only for successfully resolving the problem, but additionally for *your efforts*. This an important point, in that regardless of the results of your efforts concerning any one problem, by trying to put your problem-solving skills to work and monitoring the results, you will always be improving your skills, regardless of the outcome. For instance, in the example above, Jane was mostly pleased with her overall performance but was somewhat disappointed that her boss was going to increase her salary only 10%, rather than the 20% she requested. Although Jane rated her satisfaction at the overall results as "somewhat satisfactory," she indicated that she learned "a whole lot" about herself and how, over the years, at work and at home, she had "given off the vibe that I wouldn't ask for much in return for my dedication and hard work and often sold myself short." This led to a commitment to be more honest and assert herself in the future, rather than always passively take what other people gave her, only to resent them later. As such, she gained a lot more by solving this problem than simply getting a raise.

## TROUBLESHOOT AREAS OF DIFFICULTY

We believe that when first trying to put problem-solving skills into practice, like any new set of skills, we find ourselves making a few mistakes and needing to circle back through our efforts to determine what we could have done to improve the effectiveness of our problem solving. Think of what it was like when you learned a new skill. It is important when trying to develop new skills that we observe ourselves and self-monitor our performance it order to improve them. Whether it is something we are learning in school, business, sports, parenting, hobbies such as cooking, photography, or playing a musical instrument, practice, self-monitoring, and making adjustments are important steps to take to becoming competent. Only by practicing and monitoring ourselves can we identify the areas that are in need of the most practice.

For example, as Jane reviewed her office behavior over the past few years, she realized that she often wanted the approval of others, such that she would never say no to anyone, even though the demands were unreasonable. As a result, people asked more and more of her without providing compensation. As she circled back through her problem-solving efforts, she realized that in defining the problem, she was making many false assumptions that people would eventually recognize her work and that their approval would translate into a financial reward. She understood that this was not realistic—most people in her office were more likely to be focused on their own compensation packages, no matter how much they liked her.

## KNOW WHEN TO GET PROFESSIONAL HELP

When you monitor and evaluate your problem-solving efforts, you may find yourself troubleshooting the same type of obstacles that are impinging on your problem-solving efforts over and over again. When this happens, it is useful to seek additional professional help. Knowing when you should seek professional help with your problem-solving efforts can be difficult. We know that in and of itself, this is an important decision or problem to solve. In general, we have found that if you experience any one or more of the following symptoms, despite trying hard to use all of the steps we have outlined in this book, seeking professional help may be a good idea.

- *Continued* feelings of hopelessness.
- *Continued* thoughts of harming yourself or others.
- Any self-destructive behavior that places you or others in danger.
- Inability to focus on problem solving due to mental confusion, inability to sustain even short periods of attention, or intruding thoughts that block your ability to complete problem-solving steps.
- Noticing that the same internal obstacles *continue* to persist (for example, negative thoughts about yourself, overwhelming emotions, or continued conflict over goals and values).

For example, Jane realized that she required some additional help in understanding why she had always formed relationships at work and in her personal life with people who exploited her willingness to take responsibility for their own work and problems. She met with a counselor for a number of sessions and learned that she had developed this pattern as a way of hoping to control how others felt about her. Beginning with her own family, Jane learned that one way she could influence others to give her approval and love was by pushing aside her own needs and taking care of everyone else's responsibilities. Having these insights was helpful to her to better understand why she made so many internal and self-critical statements to herself when she instead wanted to put her energies into her own goals. As a result, she often took care of everyone else and then felt abandoned and angry when they were not supportive of what she wanted for herself. Knowing this helped her to work hard to catch herself in the act of engaging in these behaviors. As such, Jane eventually was able to feel better about herself and went on to improve her relationships with people at work.

## CONGRATULATIONS!

You learned the five steps to becoming an effective problem solver. In the next and last chapter, as an additional aid, we provide examples of how to apply these five steps to various common problems.

# CHAPTER 9

# Applying the Five Steps of Effective Problem Solving to Common Life Problems

## LEARNING BY EXAMPLE

Up until now, we have provided you with specific instructions and suggestions regarding ways in which to improve your problem-solving skills by using our step-by-step guide. In this final chapter, we offer some examples of how people we have worked with have used the five steps of effective problem solving in their everyday lives in order to adapt to stressful life difficulties. The challenge in doing so, as we have indicated many times throughout this guide, is to provide such examples while continuing to underscore the idea that *what represents an effective or useful solution for one person, at one point in their life, is not the same solution that will be best for someone else.*

For instance, imagine asking a football coach the following question—"What is the one best play to use when you want to score a touchdown?" This would be an impossible question to answer. All football coaches and players know that it would depend on *many* factors, unique to the particular situation, such as field position, time left in the game, skills and personality of the other team, current weather conditions, number of injured players, level of fatigue, and so forth.

What does this football analogy have to do with problem solving? Actually, very much! There is no one right solution to any given human problem. There are, however, ways in which people can be effective problem solvers who, like expert coaches, know how to keep up team spirit and an optimistic outlook, analyze a situation, define the problem, think creatively, weigh all the potential options, design a play, and then implement it. They also know how to review and evaluate a play to see if the outcome was what they anticipated. Although coaches may not be able to tell you exactly what to do in a given situation, they can often provide examples by taking the listener step-by-step through their decision-making process. This is what we chose to do as a way of providing you with examples—have individuals who have become effective problem solvers that we worked with (Catherine, Jim, Tad, and Mary) relate personal stories of how they used their newly learned problem-solving skills to help them adapt to and cope better with difficult life problems. Their problem-solving stories will be related to you in the first person, as they take you through the ways in which they each used *ADAPT* to solve a difficult problem. We ask that you pay special attention to *how* they used the skills provided in this guidebook, rather than *what* they actually did in one situation, at one specific point in time.

## PROBLEM AREAS

We asked our problem solvers to describe how they navigated a tough problem that resulted in their experience of depressive, anxious, or angry symptoms. These three emotions are often the reason for which people seek counseling or psychotherapy, and although many life problems and situations are associated with these symptoms, taking a well-practiced problem-solving approach can often help the symptoms to improve as substantial research continues to document. We will introduce each person's story with an description of the problem they decided to tackle.

## CATHERINE'S PROBLEM: LONELINESS AND DEPRESSION

One of the frequent problems that people report concerns the pain of being alone. Many times a crisis or situation in life serves as a trigger for feelings of loneliness and depression. This might include the breakup of a long-term relationship, the move to a new residence, aging, grown children leaving the home, unemployment, or an illness or disability that isolates us from other people. Although all of these situations have different characteristics, loneliness is a frequent problem for which one can practice their new problem-solving skills. In the following description, Catherine, a 64-year old woman who was divorced from her husband 10 years prior, provides a description of her experience and how she put her skills into action when tackling this difficult problem. Here is her story:

## MY STORY

I had been feeling real sad and down for quite a bit of time. In particular, I felt very lonely. I loved my house, but sometimes it seems to be so empty and so big. I just didn't know what to do. I used to be so full of life and energy, especially when the kids were small. I missed my kids—it's too bad that they had to move to other parts of the country. I just didn't know what to do. I was encouraged by one of my daughters to go to see a counselor. I initially thought that was crazy—I was just lonely, not "out of my mind!" But she told me to see someone who would work with me and teach me some skills to help me cope better. Because she was a social worker, she had some information about who to see that was close to my home. I was scared to go in the therapist's office, but he explained that he was going to teach me "problem-solving skills" to help me come up with my own plan, just as if I was going to a cooking class or painting class—he was going to be more of a teacher than anything else. This approach made me feel better.

### Adopting a Positive Problem-Solving Attitude

I was initially taught to try to adopt a positive problem-solving attitude. This led me to tell myself that loneliness and sadness were, in fact, common human experiences. Because I was experiencing the feelings of depression and pain that come with loneliness, it did not mean there was anything wrong with me or that I am the only person who ever felt this way. I decided that I could realistically do some things to improve my experience of loneliness, but recognized that it would take some time and effort and there were no perfect solutions that could completely remove my feelings of being lonely—but they could be reduced.

### Defining the Problem

First, I started a fresh journal and thought about the situations in which I most experienced a sense of loneliness. I took the role of a news reporter by asking myself the questions "who, what, when, where, why, and how." I discovered that I felt most painfully alone and sad on weekends. The most accurate explanation I could figure out when I looked objectively at the situation was that my children had all grown and moved out of the immediate area. Weekends were usually taken up in the past with family activities—now I had so much free time on the weekends without any real plans. I often ended up calling my grown children who were generally kind and supportive, but I knew that they had their own work and families that required their time. After such conversations, I would start to have thoughts that my usefulness as a person was over. Next, I thought about my goal. Although I would love to have back some of the years in which I was raising my family, I realized that it was not possible, and the truth was, I currently had few friends and very little sense of purpose in my life. Therefore, I knew that I should develop a realistic goal of meeting two new people with whom I could plan a few weekend activities in the next few months.

Next, I thought about what was standing in my way or blocking the path to my goal. I realized that before I even gave an idea a chance, I had a tendency to think of all the things that could go wrong. What if I didn't like the new people I met. Worse yet, what if they didn't like me? Because I was a homemaker most of my life, and had few formally trained skills, what if I couldn't find any purposeful activities on the weekend?

In defining my problem, I realized that I had a strong tendency to be a "worrier" about everything. I listed a secondary goal of trying out some new alternatives in spite of my worries (especially if my worries were bigger than they had to be!). For example, throughout my life, many people have said they enjoyed my company and I have enjoyed the company of others. There was an equal chance of being liked or liking others, as much as there was a chance that we would not like each other. This next part was tough for me to face—as I thought about feeling bad over not having a strong purpose in life, I asked myself why I only felt this way now? Then it hit me ... I had a strong sense of purpose when I was raising children. It might not make sense to try to discover some *general* life purpose, but to think of *current* goals as my life purpose. This part of trying to better understand my problems was important because it helped me to see my current goals as very important to my life *right now!*

## Generating Alternative Solutions

Next, I generated a bunch of alternative solutions according to those brainstorming rules, trying to be as creative as possible, and especially important for me (who tends to be a worrier), to not be judgmental. In terms of my goal of meeting two new people with whom I can make some weekend plans, I generated the following list:

- Sign up for a cooking or foreign language class at the senior center
- Join a gym
- Volunteer to help at the church
- Volunteer to help at the animal shelter
- Join a community choir
- Join a support group for retirees

- Put an ad in the newspaper
- Join a discussion group on the Internet
- Work for a political cause such as AARP

At times, when I felt "stuck," I thought about a role model of mine, former President Jimmy Carter, and tried to picture what alternatives he would come up with.

## Predicting Potential Consequences and Developing a Solution Plan

Next, I rated each of these alternatives according to the following criteria: likelihood that I could actually do it, likelihood that I would like the people I met through the activity or that they would like me, the costs involved (I had very little money in my budget to spend), and the overall convenience. Because I live in a city, I didn't want to have to travel very far away. After rating all of the alternatives, I chose volunteering for a church activity as one that had the most predictable positive consequences and the least amount of negative consequences.

The activity I volunteered for was to cook for the church's soup kitchen every Tuesday afternoon. This church worked with other churches in the area to provide meals to the homeless and gave me the opportunity to meet new people from this affiliated church.

## Trying Out My Solution Choice With an Action Plan

One of the reasons why I chose this solution had to do with it being very cost-effective and also pretty easy to carry out. I had to sign up for the Tuesday afternoon time slot and show up with my sleeves rolled up and ready to cook. I had some skill as a cook, so this activity had the added bonus of feeling good about myself.

## Rating the Outcome

After working for three Tuesdays, I met a woman from the other church who loved good food and wine as much as I did. We decided to take ourselves out for a nice dinner and movie on the weekend. We had such a nice time that we are now discussing the possibility of starting a "movie and dinner" club for older single women in our two churches. Some surprises that occurred when I looked back in hindsight was how much energy I put into feeling sorry for myself being lonely, sad, and worried about not having a purpose in life, that it actually kept me from trying to meet new people and discovering my day-to-day, moment-to-moment purpose. I can now say that my current purpose in life is to help less fortunate people, make good meals, and be a good friend to some of the women I have met recently. Not all will work perfectly, but some will result in a better quality of life for me. Isn't that what it's all about?

## JIM'S PROBLEM: COMMITTING TO HEALTHY BEHAVIOR HABITS

Many times people seek counseling for help in changing their behavior in order to develop healthier lifestyle habits. Sometimes their interest is somewhat cosmetic, such as wanting to shed unwanted pounds or to improve their self-esteem. Other times, however, they are referred by their physician to help change behavior habits that are directly or indirectly impacting their health and medical status. For example, changing diet and exercise regimens is often prescribed by patients' doctors to better manage significant medical conditions like diabetes, high blood pressure, various allergies, and clinical obesity. In addition, doctors are increasingly concerned about the role emotions play, such as anger, anxiety, and depression, in worsening medical vulnerabilities. Many patients have been referred to us by their doctors in order to learn how to better manage the stress in their lives, as well as learning non-pharmaceutical alternatives for reducing chronic pain or treating insomnia. However, many of the techniques used by behavioral medicine professionals to treat most problems related to changing behavior require that a patient remain motivated and committed to the behavior change strategies that are suggested. In the example below, Jim tells us how he used his problem-solving skills to remain committed to changing his diet and exercise regimen when he was diagnosed with type 2 diabetes and high cholesterol. Here is his story:

## MY STORY

When I first learned that I had diabetes, I felt as though my whole world had changed for the worst. I come from a big Italian family, where eating pasta, drinking wine, and homemade desserts are all part of the love and good times of family life. I felt alone and scared, even though I was always a pretty tough guy. I couldn't imagine having trouble with my heart, vision, and circulation, all potential problems if my diabetes continued to remain uncontrolled. I learned about how to use problem solving to help me make the changes I need to make because one of my best friends is a nurse and she gave me a guidebook on problem solving.

## Adopting a Positive Problem-Solving Attitude

When I took the self-assessment test, I was pretty surprised at my scores. I always thought of myself as a good problem solver. I work in construction, and unless you can always be ready for the unexpected and be creative about ideas on how to fix things, you would be in deep trouble! Although I did have some strong points, such as being creative, I also found out on this test just how cynical and pessimistic I am. Other than construction problems, I tend to see other kinds of problems as too big to handle, having no good answers, and as a result, I frequently just leave or withdraw from problems. When I talked to my wife about my high score for a "negative problem-solving attitude," she said it was because I was such a "perfectionist." In my work, I can usually find a near-perfect solution (finding the "right tool for the right job"), but for other problems, if I can't fix something, my usual response is "screw it" and I give up. It was tough to learn this about myself, but if I wanted to get better at solving other kinds of problems, I would have to be less of a perfectionist and a little more accepting of life problems not being all neat and tidy, just like my construction jobs.

## Defining the Problem

I knew it was important to start exercising on a regular basis and to reduce my blood sugar level by reducing the number of carbohydrates and sugars in my diet. At first, I did well. Right after my diagnosis, I educated myself about diets, started a medication that my doctor prescribed, and signed up for a membership in a local gym. My blood glucose dropped to close to normal range! Over time, however, after my initial weight loss and some success in lowering my blood glucose levels, I found myself less likely to go the gym because of time constraints and grabbing fast food meals when under pressure at work. My glucose readings were starting to be more unpredictable and I was feeling like a failure for not "fixing" the problem correctly. Wow, my wife was really right about me wanting to give up when I can't fix things perfectly! I tried really hard to adjust my attitude to be more realistic. This idea made sense to me and it is what I would say to a good friend who was going through a similar situation. I just had to learn to take my own advice. I listed my goals and obstacles as follows:

## Goals:

- To keep my motivation up
- To maintain a low-carbohydrate, low-sugar diet
- To exercise at least 30 minutes each day

## Obstacles:

- I often rush from the house in the morning and have trouble thinking about what to have for breakfast, so I often miss breakfast.
- Work schedules make it difficult to get to the gym.
- I look forward to my favorite television shows.
- I enjoy the time I spend in the early evening reading to my three-year-old daughter and I am too tired to work out afterward.

### Generating Alternative Solutions

This is the part of problem solving that I am good at—coming up with ideas about how to solve a problem. I knew that if I tried to reach all my goals at once, I might be setting myself up for failure. That's probably a good example of how my tendency to try and fix everything worked *against* me. So, I further separated my goals into both a dietary goal and a workout goal. I decided to work on the dietary goal first. Breakfast was often missed because I did not have the time to make decisions and prepare breakfast before leaving the house before my 30-minute drive to work. I came up with a creative list of ideas that included both strategies and tactics.

- Make breakfast the night before
- Buy prepackaged breakfasts
- Eat a breakfast snack bar on the way to work
- Ask for help from a nutritionist to prepare my meals
- Ask for advice and suggestions from a diabetes support helpline on the Internet
- Ask my wife for help to select a number of different low-carb, low-sugar breakfast alternatives when she shops and bring home samples to better know what I like.

### Predicting Potential Consequences and Developing a Solution Plan

I weighed each alternative with a series of plusses and minuses.... Many of them had very little positive consequences (most breakfast bars are high in sugar and I don't like the taste of those that are not). Several alternatives were expensive (prepackaged foods) or costly in terms of my time and money (setting up consultation from a professional nutritionist). Some had further health risks (forget the diet, eat whatever I want and ask my doctor for larger doses of medication). There were two that had the highest ratings—sample food with my wife's help, and prepare my breakfast to be eaten on the way to work at the beginning of the week. These two alternatives seemed to go well together and when combined, offered me the most positive consequences and the least negative consequences. Foods I discovered liking were a low-carb cereal, blueberries, and nuts.

## Trying Out My Solution Choice With an Action Plan

My wife and I made up packets of the cereal on Sunday in baggies, mixed with nuts and blueberries. I took a packet each day when I left for work, along with a bottle of water.

## Rating the Outcome

I discovered that I was less hungry for lunch and less likely to gobble down fast food. I actually liked my own special cereal mix and found myself looking forward to my commute and breakfast "on the road." Most of all, this was a great head start for me to realize that there are ways that I can improve my glucose management and tackle the trouble spots as they come up. I used the same principles to work on the exercise problem. The end product? A before-dinner "Gymboree" with my daughter that gave us great exercise and a time to bond each day!

## TAD'S PROBLEM: COPING WITH LOSS

Although many of us realize that change is a fact of life, it is very challenging for people to cope with change when it involves loss. The loss may involve the death of a loved one, the loss of plans and dreams through divorce, or even the loss of neighbors and a familiar environment through a geographical move. Loss can be, and often is, embedded in changes that are simultaneously happy (such as the joy experienced by parents when their children attend college) and simultaneously sad (such as the loss associated with an "empty nest"). Another example may be the relief of successful surgery or expert medical care following an accident or illness, coupled with some loss of physical functioning. Retirement can bring great opportunities for new activities and travel but can also signal the loss of power, income, and personal identity. Whether or not the loss occurs is often out of our control. The example below highlights that when problem-solving skills are applied to a problem of loss, it often starts with being able to accurately identify what losses cannot be changed and what parts of the loss can be improved through problem solving.

Tad was a 26-year-old man with bone cancer (knee). At the time of his diagnosis, he had been working for an accounting firm for about a year. He had received very positive reviews about his performance and his supervisor indicated that it was likely that he would receive a promotion in the next six months. However, the demands of his cancer treatment led to limited physical, social, and occupational functioning. He was very distressed over the loss of his limb and focused most of his concerns on the loss of his career path. In fact, he stated his initial reason for coming to treatment as, "My boss expects me to get as much work done during my three-day a week, half-time work, while I am recuperating and getting additional chemotherapy, as I did when I worked full-time." He backed up these assumptions with memos from his boss who requested status reports on jobs that he was currently working on. Here is Tad's problem-solving story:

## MY STORY

I'll be honest. At first I thought that a problem-solving self-assessment was a dumb idea. To my way of thinking, I wouldn't have any problems if I didn't have cancer. How could anyone be a "good" problem solver in a situation like this? When I looked at my answers to the test, I saw that it said that I was pretty good at defining problems and coming up with ideas about how to solve them, but that I didn't have much of a positive problem-solving attitude. This was no big surprise, but it also made me think about the fact that if I had a little more positive optimism about my ability to work in the future, maybe I could come up with some ideas about how to keep my job, rather than spend my time worrying about losing it. I also realized that I was making a whole lot of assumptions about why my boss requested status reports about my job. I immediately thought that he was looking for information that he would use to fire me, but I really didn't have any proof of that.

### Adopting a Positive Problem-Solving Attitude

I decided to post some of the "healthy thinking rules" on my refrigerator to remind myself to think more positively. I particularly liked the sayings that talked about having a choice in the way that you think about things.

I started to make a list of positive experiences in my life, along with the loss. I had great medical care and I had a group of guys (my poker buddies) that I knew since college who stuck by me through this whole thing. I had some really "cool people" in my family. My dad and mom are divorced and I don't see my dad much, but my mom was an amazing source of support. I still had a job (even though I thought that I had no chance at the promotion), and I actually had some good benefits so I could take the time to recuperate.

## Defining the Problem

I laid out the problem. I needed to work less hours, but the obstacle was that my boss wanted me to work the same hours I always did in order to get the promotion in six months. When I followed the problem-solving advice to separate out facts from assumptions, I had a talk with my boss (which I initially rehearsed with my buddies), in which I asked him about his specific expectations and the impact of my cancer on the chances of me getting that promotion. I was shocked to hear from him that he did *not* expect me to work the same hours, and that my promotion could be reconsidered six months after I returned to work full-time when ready! He had asked for status reports because he knew that he would need to do some reassignment of work during my recovery process and it was helpful to know the status of each client. My definition of the problem actually changed at that point, as I began to be much more interested in using problem solving to come up with the best plan to maximize my recovery. Since I live alone, this took some planning and my problem-solving efforts were now more focused on ways to get practical help getting to my cancer treatment appointments, help to shop for healthy food, and help to get me to a special yoga class for amputees at my local cancer wellness treatment center.

## Generating Alternative Solutions

I made a list of the three major activities for which I needed help, then brainstormed a list of anyone and everyone that could possibly be of help. This was a little difficult, because after I named my buddies and my mom, I felt stuck. I thought about the ways that my problem-solving counselor taught me to get "unstuck," such as imagining that someone I admire had to come up with additional people for the list. I asked my buddies during a poker game to help me add to the list (following all the rules of not judging any alternatives). I turned it into a game and told them I would buy dinner for the one who came up with the most people to add to the list. Wow! Was that helpful! In addition to the five of them and my mom, the list included people from the Jewish community center where my mom volunteers, the people I work with, the rotary club (one of my clients was a long-time member), an ad in the paper, a flyer in my doctor's office, and some people at the yoga class.

## Predicting Potential Consequences and Developing a Solution Plan

With so many choices, this was pretty easy to weigh the pros and cons of the different ways I could ask people to help me with my rehabilitation process. I used criteria that focused on my personal values, such as how comfortable I would be with the person helping me, and consideration of ways to express my appreciation. The final list had 20 people who were willing to roll up their sleeves and pitch in to bring me to appointments, shopping, and yoga class!

## Trying Out My Solution Choice With an Action Plan

It's a good thing that I work as an accountant, because it took some management skills to organize all the volunteers that resulted from the list that was developed (and later rated through the decision-making process) from my brainstorming session. I made a big calendar to keep track of what was happening each day and who would be helping me. I kept in touch with everyone by e-mail. Each evening I would confirm the appointment for the next day.

## Rating the Outcome

I was able to increase the quality of my recovery process with the additional practical help. I also got some unexpected results. As you might imagine, I developed additional friends and supports that I am close with to this day. I also realized that my whole initial focus was on feeling hopeless about the loss of my leg and seeing it as "ruining" my chances for a career future. This was a huge overexaggeration. The truth is, my loss actually delayed (versus "ruined") my career path, and the time out from my career incidentally made me realize how important my friends were.

## MARY'S PROBLEM: ANGER WITH PEOPLE WHO "PUSH MY BUTTONS"

One of the most common problems that people seek treatment for is help with managing their interactions with others. This can involve an inattentive or insensitive spouse or partner, an intrusive and guilt-inducing parent, or a friend who has behaved in ways that are hurtful, bullying, or hostile.

When we are in the middle of an interpersonal situation in which someone is pushing our buttons, we often experience a surge of emotion in which we feel powerless to manage our reactions, out of control, and unable to effectively respond. As one of our patients described it, when caught in difficult interpersonal situations, she often felt like a "deer caught in the headlights." This is a very apt analogy as we often feel surprised, frozen, and emotionally (if not physically) in danger of being significantly hurt.

Mary is a 48-year-old woman, who described herself as being "under my parents' thumb" her whole life. Her parents, who were now in their 70s, had managed to have Mary and her brother Jack always close to home. Mary had a history of problem relationships with men who had been abusive to her. She described her parents as always reminding her that "blood is thicker than water" and reiterated this philosophy when Mary had divorced her abusive husband over 20 years previously. More recently, Mary had met a man with whom she shared much in common and one who had understood and experienced being the victim of physical abuse. He realized, long ago, through therapy, that his own experience with a depressed and violent father had contributed to his low self-confidence and provided him with little help in learning to cope with various stresses and strains of life. When he and Mary started to date, and continuing after they married, she was often surprised and hurt that her parents stated their strong disapproval when she would not put them first in terms of all of her time, energy, and love. They frequently placed her in a position of choosing between them and her new husband (stating, for example, "How can you go out with your husband and friends when we need you to take us to a doctor's appointment?"). In addition, Mary's brother also criticized her and feared that he would now be called upon to provide some caretaking of their parents. Soon Mary and her new husband, Frank, were getting into arguments. Protective of Mary, Frank would voice his disapproval of Mary's parents and indicate that she needed to react differently for the sake of their marriage. Mary, caught in conflict, worry, and self-doubt, often wished that Frank would just let her do whatever would get them "to stop pushing my buttons," even if that meant sacrificing her own wishes or happiness. Mary and Frank came to therapy to get some help with the situation. The toughest part of applying problem solving in this case was for Mary to adopt a realistic problem orientation that she could make positive changes in her life. Here is Mary's story:

## MY STORY

I read many self-help books and watched television shows like "Dr. Phil" and "Oprah" as a way of trying to get answers to my problem, but I was experiencing the same problem over and over again. One day, I blacked out and fainted. When my husband brought me to the emergency room, my doctor performed many tests and referred me to a neurologist. The doctors finally told me that they had no medical explanation for the fainting episode and suggested that it might be due to stress. That is when I realized that I needed help. My therapist had me take a problem-solving test and discussed the results with me. She said that I had very little confidence in my ability to solve day-to-day problems so I usually avoided them, and that I had a strong tendency to feel particularly trapped and hopeless about problems that I experience with my family.

## Adopting a Positive Problem-Solving Attitude

I sought out help from a therapist because I was having such anxiety about dealing with my family problems and my husband was worried about my physical health. He said that he was helped in the past by a therapist who taught him different ways to think and change certain habits that were self-destructive. I was nervous and shaking when I walked into the therapist's office because I knew that I would have to make some changes in my life if I wanted to help myself and my marriage.

## Defining the Problem

My problem was pretty clear—how to put limits on the demands that my parents and brother were making on me without feeling so guilty and worried when I have to say no. I wanted to tell my parents that I loved them and want to be of help, but there are times when I can't be present because of my work and plans that I make with my husband. The big obstacle was that when they "pushed my guilt buttons," I started to feel a sense of panic about doing something wrong. I realized that these feelings were very exaggerated, because my parents were robust seniors, had resources, and were there for each other. One big obstacle was that I had been taught not to trust anyone other than my family, and my first husband, who was physically abusive, seemed to provide "proof" that this was true. However, the facts of my current marriage were different. My husband, Frank, was very caring and respectful of what I wanted, more than anyone I had known. My parents and brother were behaving in ways that were very immature, getting angry and having tantrums when they didn't get their way. I was trying to change them and at the same time keep them happy 100% of the time … an impossible expectation.

## Generating Alternative Solutions

Here is the list of alternative solutions that I generated with the therapist's help:

- Use the thinking techniques provided by the therapist to help me think more positively and rationally about my right to a marriage and a personal life that is separate from my parents.
- Tell my parents that I love them and will do what I can.
- Try to convince my parents to change.
- Move across the country (or out of the country) to get away from my parents.
- Not talk to Frank about the problems with my parents.
- Ask Frank's help in changing the way I react to my parents.
- Join a support group about how to deal with aging parents.
- Break down the problems with my parents into the smaller, day-to-day decisions.

## Predicting the Consequences

In looking at the various alternatives, the last alternative I wrote down really hit home. I realized that since I was feeling like this problem was so big and overwhelming, it would be important to first break down the problem of setting limits with my parents into smaller ones, dealing with one situation at a time. I rated this alternative as an important first step that I could then combine with some of the others. I chose a family event (a wedding shower) that my mother wanted me to take her to in the coming month. Frank and I had planned to be away at that time in the Outer Banks of North Carolina with friends. My mother wanted me to travel north in order to take her to the wedding shower, but I wanted to keep the plans I made with my husband and friends. After reviewing the other alternatives, I realized that my parents were not likely to change their way of thinking. I would have to work hard at accepting this and changing my own exaggerated guilt and worry reaction to their unfair demands. Knowing this helped me to circle back and redefine my problem a bit to be focused on how to help me reduce my exaggerated guilt reaction and to use this situation as practice for the future. I generated some additional alternatives that included asking Frank to stay calm and help me to work out what to say (I noticed that when he became angry at my parents, it made me feel worse). In addition, I worked with my therapist to be able to use self-statements that I could tell myself whenever I started to feel guilty. These statements were based on facts and helped me work against the years of guilty and unfair self-criticism I had learned over the years.

## Trying Out My Solution Choice With an Action Plan

I told my parents that I loved them, but that there are times that I couldn't always do what they wanted. I was careful not to try and convince them that it was wrong to make such demands, because that usually led to an argument and I had to accept that they would not always be 100% pleased with my decisions. I asked Frank to practice with me, and this was helpful because he knew the things that my parents would say to "push my buttons." I practiced saying various self-statements silently to myself that I prepared with my therapist in order to hit the "off button" when my parents started in on me. I had a helpful alternative prepared in which I offered to help my mother think about who else could take her to the shower. After several minutes of complaining, she agreed to call a cousin to take her.

## Rating the Outcome

I was very uncomfortable initially, but when I started to see how manipulative my parents had been, I realized that I was actually contributing to the problem by not thinking more realistically and always self-sacrificing. I also came to trust Frank's support and help and my marriage has never been better. My parents still complain and believe that my brother and I should always be ready to drop everything at their whim, but I am working on accepting that they are not going to change. As a result, I experience much less guilt and panic, my brother and I are closer, and they are not able to push my buttons as much anymore.

## FINAL THOUGHTS

- A major theme throughout this guidebook involved the need to practice the problem-solving skills similar to any other sport, hobby, or new skill that you are learning. We wish to emphasize that point once again as a reminder. As the 13th-century Persian philosopher, Sa'di, stated (our paraphrase)—"However much you read in theory, if you do not practice, you remain in the dark."
- In going through this guidebook, you probably wondered whether we advocate that you go through each of the five steps each time you have a stressful problem. *Absolutely not!* Instead, we hope, through practice, that by using these skills, they eventually become automatic and applied with greater ease. However, you might find that some problems require additional time and effort to define accurately, whereas others necessitate additional effort focused on making a difficult decision. Still others require a larger list of possible solutions or a more complex solution plan. We suggest that you apply those skills that are required by a particular situation. You will know when to do so if you

follow the guidelines outlined in Chapter 5 regarding how to recognize problems. In other words, use your feelings, thoughts, and behavior as guides to help you realize when you need to engage more vigorously in a particular problem-solving skill. However, as mentioned previously, many of our patients have indicated that what has helped them the most is having such a guidebook to go back to and use the step-by-step approach when faced with a particularly difficult problem.

- There might be occasions in the future when you need to solve a problem within a limited period of time. To help you meet this challenge, we provide a "rapid problem-solving guide" in the appendix.
- You probably noticed that we enjoyed providing quotes throughout this guidebook as a means of emphasizing or illustrating various points. In this same spirit, we would like to end with a quote by Helen Keller, the woman who struggled with becoming deaf and blind due to a childhood illness, and who eventually came to be a role model for her charity work to millions of people. We feel her statement sums up the philosophy of this book:

> All the world is full of suffering;
> It is also full of overcoming it.

# Appendices

# A. Visualization for Success Exercise

The following exercise can help you to lay out various problem-solving goals and feel more motivated to try to attain them. It asks you to use your imagination in order to "travel to the future" and visit yourself several years from now. In this visualization, anything goes—so picture it just the way that you want it to be. You will be asked to look around at your surroundings and your possessions, notice your accomplishments, see who you are with, be aware of how you spend your leisure time, and so forth.

Below is a script that contains specific instructions for this visualization exercise. We suggest that either you or a friend make a tape recording of this script in order to practice the exercise at home. In doing so, be sure to read slowly, pausing at places where you are being asked to concentrate and think of a certain image. Try to visualize a scene as well as possible, using your *mind's eye* and all of your other senses. Try to *experience* the situation as best you can. By recording it, you can listen at your leisure and not have to be distracted by trying to remember what is being asked of you. We include the actual script for your information.

## VISUALIZATION SCRIPT

Close your eyes and relax—let go of any tension in your body. Now go to a safe and tranquil place in your mind—a special, outdoor place. Look around, take note of what you see nearby, as well as in the distance. Describe the scene silently to yourself. Now look for a path—this is your path toward the future. Notice a tree stump or log branch across the path. Imagine that this piece of wood in front of the path is getting in the way of your ability to walk down the path. This piece of wood is your own hesitation or fear of changing and walking toward your goals. Step over it, step over this log and visualize overcoming your hesitation, overcoming your fears.

Now, as you walk along the path, you come across a steep hill. This hill is your own doubts about yourself. Slowly keep walking up the hill, even though you are not absolutely sure of what you will find at the top of the hill. With each step, begin to let yourself become more self-confident that you will reach your goals.

When you reach the top, you walk through a dark forest of trees that block out the sunlight. This forest has *all* the obstacles that block you from seeing your final goals—interference from others, day-to-day problems that keep you from working on your goals, or your own fears that you don't deserve what you want. However, you push past the trees to a clearing and you are now in a sunny field. You can see your home in the distance. This is your home several years in the future where you feel safe and peaceful.

Go into your home and look around. What do you see? How is it decorated? What pictures or photographs do you see? Look at yourself in the mirror. What do you look like? Notice that your family or friends are entering the room. How do they act toward each other? Listen to yourself as you interact with others—what makes you experience joy? What are the achievements you are most proud of? In your free time, what are you doing? For example, maybe you're watching TV, race-car driving, sailing, fishing, playing with children, or listening to classical music.

Now ask yourself—what are you most grateful for? In other words, looking back over the last few years, what are you especially glad that you had the chance to experience? What are you most proud of? Maybe you gave a successful speech, ran a marathon, had several good friends, raised self-confident children, visited a sick friend, or people knew that they could count on you. Anything is possible. Remember—visualize what you hope and wish to be in the future—not what is going on now!

When you have finished exploring, let your images fade away and come back to the present—here and now. Open your eyes and make a brief list with your images still fresh in your mind. Pick one or two major goals for your future and write down the details and the specific visual images that come to mind.

## CREATE A WEEKLY VISUALIZATION

Create a visualization once a week in order to plan your specific steps toward these goals. In your imagination, picture yourself clearly carrying out the steps for your immediate goals. For example, picture yourself exercising two days per week for the next four months. Visualize yourself in your workout clothes, imagining that you will experience a sense of pride in arranging for enough time to spend at the gym. Imagine your favorite music playing on your personal tape player and visualize your body feeling strong and the perspiration dripping off your skin. It is likely that every time you visualize this sequence, you will *experience* the positive effects of reaching your goals and will be able to make a stronger commitment to actually do it.

Alternatively, visualize being able to see a live professional football game. Visualize saving $5 a week by giving up a second cup of coffee during your commute to work—watch your football fund build up. Visualize learning how to use the computer to search the Web for tickets. Imagine being able to get two tickets on the 40-yard line!

Alternatively, visualize yourself living in a home where you experience a sense of warmth and safety and freedom from debt. Visualize having other people to love and support you in this home. Visualize getting to this goal by first having a temporary move to a shared apartment, where you are able to cut your current housing expenses in half, working with a financial consultant from the local bank, asking friends and family to help you search out potential living arrangements where you might have close geographical access to visit, and learning about the costs and benefits of all possible living alternatives (for example, rentals, single homes, condominiums, retirement communities).

Alternatively, visualize your own set of goals. As you reach each goal that you have visualized, begin weekly, and even daily, visualizations of the steps to take to reach additional goals.

By now, we hope that we have illustrated that the best reason to use the basic strategy of visualizing future goals is so that you can develop a "road map" of steps that you need to take to achieve such goals. In developing this road map, write down overall goals, as well as smaller steps leading to these goals. When we are thinking about a goal that seems far away, it is often difficult to maintain the patience required to focus on the final goal. This is why many people give up on their goals—because the reinforcement seems so far away. Visualizing reaching each step allows us all to have a continual stream of personal reward and recognition of progress, no matter how small, to keep us going for it.

# B. Deep Breathing Exercise to Manage Stress

This is simply to help you combat physical feelings of anxiety and tension. Like most people, you probably take breathing for granted. If so, you may not realize the "medicine" that you carry within yourself all of the time, every day. Although breathing seems to be a simple and automatic activity, *how* you breathe can have extremely important consequences for your health.

Certain types of breathing can be especially good for you. Psychologists have shown that by teaching people how to breathe slowly and regularly, they can quiet their minds by helping their bodies to relax. Further, there is scientific evidence to show that deep and rhythmic breathing can also improve the rhythms of your heart. The current scientific research suggests that the use of a combination of focused breathing and positive mental states when exposed to an emotionally stressful experience is an important method for being able to effectively offset negative mind/body reactions to daily stressors.

Breathing for your health and well-being requires you to breathe from your abdominal or stomach area. This type of breathing is also referred to as *diaphragmatic breathing* and is very different than breathing from your chest area. Chest breathing often occurs when we experience even mild stress. It is irregular, rapid, and shallow breathing. In some cases, when people are very scared or upset, they may actually hold their breath. Other people breathe so fast that they hyperventilate and can actually pass out. Breathing improperly can contribute to many problems, such as essential hypertension (that is, high blood pressure), panic attacks, muscle tension, tiredness, headaches, and negative moods.

Abdominal or deep diaphragmatic breathing, on the other hand, is the type of natural breathing we do as babies, as well as when we are relaxed and resting peacefully as adults. It is also used by singers to get the most out of their voices, and for pain management, like the panting form of breathing used by women during childbirth. Diaphragmatic breathing is one of the simplest, cheapest, and safest ways to help our bodies calm down. According to doctors who specialize in mind and body interactions, breathing is an incredibly powerful health tool that we have available to us at all times.

## DEEP BREATHING

Follow the steps below to learn how to make more effective use of your breathing for your health, as well as to better manage stress.

*Step 1.* Lie down or sit in a comfortable position and close your eyes.

*Step 2.* Place your hands gently on your body. Put your right hand on your stomach, just under your rib cage and about even with your waistline. Put your left hand on the center of your chest, just under your neck.

*Step 3.* Become aware of your breathing. Notice how you are breathing. Which hand rises the most? If the hand on your stomach or belly is moving up and down, then you are breathing more from your diaphragm or abdomen. This is the best way to breathe. Practice doing this now, keeping your hands on your belly. As you take in your breath, imagine that your entire abdomen, just below your rib cage, is a balloon that is filling up with air. When you exhale, let all the air out of the belly slowly, and feel it collapse, just like a balloon that is letting out air.

*Step 4.* Follow the breathing directions for about five minutes.

- Inhale *slowly* and *deeply* through your nose into your abdomen, filling all the spaces in your belly with air (if you have difficulty breathing through your nose, go ahead and breathe through your mouth).
- Now exhale through your mouth, making a quiet, exhaling whooshing sound like the wind, as you gently and slowly blow out. Purse your lips, forming an O, and release your breath, as if you were trying to make a paper sailboat glide *slowly* across the water. Take long slow, deep breaths.
- Feel your belly rise and fall.
- Repeat a phrase (silently or out loud) with each breath, such as "I take in life" with each breath in and "I am giving life" with each breath out (another phrase can include: "I am taking in a good breath and now I am releasing the tension").
- Continue to breathe this way for approximately five minutes.

Try to practice this breathing exercise at least once a day—it only takes three to five minutes. As you get better at this skill, you can try to use it to calm your body down during times of stress without having to close your eyes and place your hands on your stomach. It may come in handy, for example, while waiting in a long line at the supermarket, getting caught in traffic, right before a major presentation at work, or in the middle of a difficult exam. Apply this skill especially when you are feeling increased stress when attempting to solve a problem.

# C. Visualization—Travel to a Safe Place

The visualization exercise described in Chapter 5 was to help you to better see the light at the end of the tunnel whenever you begin to feel pessimistic about your chances of solving or coping with a difficult problem. This visualization exercise is more of a stress-management tool—specifically geared to help you to decrease any negative emotions or arousal. Similar to the other one, you will be asked to use your *mind's eye* to vividly imagine a scene. But this time, it will be one that represents a *safe place*, similar to a favorite vacation spot. Think of it as taking a vacation in your mind as a means of relaxing and calming your body. Your safe place is there for you to relax, feel safe and secure, let go, and completely be yourself. Under times of stress, it can be extremely helpful. This tool can also put you in a relaxed state of mind in anticipation of undergoing a stressful event (for example, asking your boss for a raise).

## PREPARATION

We suggest that either you or a friend make a tape-recording of this script in order to practice the exercise at home. In doing so, be sure to read slowly, pausing at places where you are being asked to concentrate and think of a certain image. Try to visualize the scene as well as possible, using your *mind's eye* and all of your other senses. Try to *experience* the situation as best you can. By recording it, you can listen at your leisure and not have to be distracted by trying to remember what is being asked of you. You can even add some of your own favorite relaxing instrumental music playing softly in the background. This way, you will be able to have your own visualization tape that you can use over and over again.

Find a comfortable location to practice visualization, such as a recliner, couch, bed, or soft floor covering. Remember to loosen your clothing, remove glasses or contact lenses, and lower the lights to create a more calming effect in the room environment. Practice once every day for at least one week. Practicing this tool is important—like learning any other skill (for example, driving a car, using a computer, playing a piano), the more you practice, the better you get. Trying this strategy only once or twice will not produce the kind of results that leads to significant reductions in anxiety or negative arousal. Therefore, practicing is important. A single session will take about 10 to 15 minutes to complete.

## VISUALIZATION SCRIPT

Let your eyes shut gently. You may find that rotating your eyeballs upward slightly and inward, looking toward the center of your forehead with your eyes gently closed, helps you to relax more quickly. The important thing to do is to close your eyes, because you are shutting out the world and about to start a voyage inward. Relax. It is important to getting the most out of visualization.

Now you are going to go to your safe place. Take a nice slow, deep breath. Now put your palms gently over your closed eyes and gently brush your hands over your eyes and face. Place your hands at your sides and allow your body to become relaxed all over. You are about to allow yourself to privately enter your own special place that is peaceful, comfortable, and safe. You will fill your imagination of this place with rich detail. You will experience this place close up, looking off into the distance and through all of your senses. You can also allow room for another person, such as your spouse, friend, or family member, to be with you in this place if you choose.

Your safe place may be at the end of a boardwalk leading to a beach. Sand is under your feet, the water is about 20 yards away, and seagulls, boats, and clouds are in the distance. You feel the coolness of the air as a cloud passes in front of the sun and seagulls are calling to each other. The sun is shimmering on the waves continually rolling to the shore, and there are smells of food emanating from the boardwalk.

A different safe place might be a warm, wood-paneled den, with the smell of cinnamon buns baking in the oven in the kitchen. Through a window you can see fields of tall dried corn stalks and there is a crackling fire in the fireplace. A set of candles emit the aroma of lavender and there is cup of warm tea on the table for you. You may have a different safe place than these two scenes. Take a few seconds to identify your safe place. It can be the beach or a warm house, or anywhere else. The point is that it is *your* place to go to.

Close your eyes now and get totally comfortable. Walk slowly to your safe and quiet place. Let your mind take you there. Your place can be inside or outside. But wherever it is, it is peaceful and safe. Picture letting your anxieties and worries pass. Look to the distance ... what do you see? Create a visual image of what you see in the distance. What do you smell? What do you hear? Notice what is right in front of you—reach out and touch it. How does it feel? Smell it ... listen for any pleasant sounds. Make the temperature comfortable. Be safe here—look around for a special, private spot. Feel the ground or earth under your feet—what does it feel like? Look above you. What do you see? What do you hear? What do you smell?

Now walk a bit further and stop. Reach out and touch something lightly with your fingertips. What is the texture of what you are touching? This is your special place and nothing can harm or upset you here. You can come here and relax whenever you want. Stay in this safe and peaceful place for as long as you wish, allowing yourself to breathe slowly and deeply and become relaxed all over.

Is there anyone else you wish to be with you? If so, imagine that he or she is now with you, also enjoying the peace and calm of your safe place. If not, that's fine—this is *your* vacation.

Now, slowly rise and leave your safe place by the same path or steps that you used to enter. Notice your surroundings ... say to yourself the following words—"I can relax here. This is my special place and I can come here whenever I wish."

Now slowly open your eyes and get used to your surroundings, but bring back home the nice feelings of relaxation.

# D. Rapid Problem Solving

Sometimes unexpected problems occur in life that require a quick decision and immediate action; thus, it becomes difficult to engage in the careful, deliberate problem-solving approach described in this guidebook. However, even if you have as little as one minute to solve a problem, several basic problem-solving principles can still help you to maximize your problem-solving effectiveness, even under these time-limited conditions.

The following are steps to take if confronted with a problem that requires a rapid but effective, problem-solving reaction:

*Step 1.* Make the following self-statements:

a.  Take a deep breath and calm down—stay in the moment
b.  There is no immediate catastrophe
c.  Think of this problem as a challenge
d.  I can handle it
e.  STOP and THINK

*Step 2.* Ask yourself the following questions:

a.  What's the problem? (State the discrepancy between what is and what should be.)
b.  What do I want to accomplish? (State a goal.)
c.  Why do I want to achieve this goal? (Broaden the goal, if appropriate.)

*Step 3.* Think of one solution idea; now think of a few additional alternative solutions (at least two or three).

*Step 4.* Think of the most important criteria for evaluating your solution ideas (at least two or three; for example, will it achieve my goal? What effect will it have on others? How much time and effort will it take? Think of any other important criteria).

a.  Decide quickly on the solution alternative that seems best.
b.  Think of one or two quick ways to improve the solution.

*Step 5.* Carry out your action plan and ask the following question:

a.  Are you satisfied with the outcome?
b.  If not, try out your second choice if you still have time.

If you find it difficult to apply the above model in three minutes or less, you can reduce the time further by eliminating Step 2c and Step 4b. Without these steps, the model may still increase the effectiveness of your problem solving under severe time pressure.

# Bibliography

The following scholarly references served as resources for this book. Many of these sources provide the scientific evidence for the five problem-solving steps.

D'Zurilla, T. J. (1990). Problem-solving training for effective stress management and prevention. *Journal of Cognitive Psychotherapy: An International Quarterly, 4,* 327–355.

D'Zurilla, T. J., & Goldfried, M. R. (1971). Problem solving and behavior modification. *Journal of Abnormal Psychology, 78,* 107–126.

D'Zurilla, T. J., & Maydeu-Olivares, A. (1995). Conceptual and methodological issues in social problem-solving assessment. *Behavior Therapy, 26,* 409–432.

D'Zurilla, T. J., & Nezu, A. M. (1982). Social problem solving in adults. In P. C. Kendall (Ed.), *Advances in cognitive-behavioral research and therapy* (Vol. 1, pp. 202–274). New York: Academic Press.

D'Zurilla, T. J., & Nezu, A. M. (1990). Development and preliminary evaluation of the Social Problem-Solving Inventory (SPSI). *Psychological Assessment: A Journal of Consulting and Clinical Psychology, 2,* 156–163.

D'Zurilla, T. J., & Nezu, A. M. (in press). *Problem-solving therapy: A positive approach to clinical intervention* (3rd ed.). New York: Springer Publishing Co.

D'Zurilla, T. J., Nezu, A. M., & Maydeu-Olivares, A. (2002). *Manual for the Social Problem-Solving Inventory-Revised.* North Tonawanda, NY: Multi-Health Systems.

D'Zurilla, T. J., Nezu, A. M., & Maydeu-Olivares, A. (2004). Social problem solving: Theory and assessment. In E. C. Chang, T. J. D'Zurilla, & L. J. Sanna (Eds.), *Social problem solving: Theory, research, and training* (pp. 11–27). Washington, DC: American Psychological Association.

Frankl, V. E. (1984). *Man's search for meaning.* New York: Pocket Books.

Levine, M. (1988). *Effective problem solving.* Englewood Cliffs, NJ: Prentice Hall.

Nezu, A. M. (2004). Problem solving and behavior therapy revisited. *Behavior Therapy, 35,* 1–33.

Nezu, A. M., D'Zurilla, T. J., Zwick, M. L., & Nezu, C. M. (2004). Problem-solving therapy for adults. In E. C. Chang, T. J. D'Zurilla, & L. J. Sanna (Eds.), *Social problem solving: Theory, research, and training* (pp. 171–191). Washington, DC: American Psychological Association.

Nezu, C. M., & Nezu, A. M. (2003). *Awakening self-esteem: Psychological and spiritual techniques for improving your well-being.* Oakland, CA: New Harbinger.

Nezu, A. M., & Nezu, C. M. (in press). Problem solving. In W. T. O'Donohue & E. Livens (Eds.), *Promoting treatment adherence: A practical handbook for health care providers.* New York: Sage Publications.

Nezu, A. M., Nezu, C. M., Friedman, S. H., Faddis, S., & Houts, P. S. (1998). *Helping cancer patients cope: A problem-solving approach.* Washington, DC: American Psychological Association.

Nezu, A. M., Nezu, C. M., Felgoise, S. H., McClure, K. S., & Houts, P. S. (2003). Project Genesis: Assessing the efficacy of problem-solving therapy for distressed adult cancer patients. *Journal of Consulting and Clinical Psychology, 71,* 1036–1048.

Nezu, A. M., Nezu, C. M., & Jain, D. (2005). *The emotional wellness way to cardiac health: How letting go of depression, anxiety, and anger can heal your heart.* Oakland, CA: New Harbinger.

Nezu, A. M., Nezu, C. M., & Perri, M. G. (1989). *Problem-solving therapy for depression: Therapy, research, and clinical guidelines.* New York: Wiley.

Nezu, A. M., & Perri, M. G. (1989). Social problem solving therapy for unipolar depression: An initial dismantling investigation. *Journal of Consulting and Clinical Psychology, 57,* 408–413.

Nezu, A. M., Wilkins, V. M., & Nezu, C. M. (2004). Social problem solving, stress, and negative affective conditions. In E. C. Chang, T. J. D'Zurilla, & L. J. Sanna (Eds.), *Social problem solving: Theory, research, and training* (pp. 49–65). Washington, DC: American Psychological Association.

Nezu, C. M., Palmatier, A., & Nezu, A. M. (2004). Social problem-solving training for caregivers. In E. C. Chang, T. J. D'Zurilla, & L. J. Sanna (Eds.), *Social problem solving: Theory, research, and training* (pp. 223–238). Washington, DC: American Psychological Association.

# Index